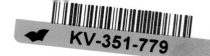

WHAT NEXT?

To Gavin, Clemency and Toby who went away and played
somewhere else, my love and thanks.

WHAT NEXT?

Post-basic Opportunities for Nurses

Jill Baker

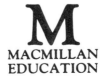

MACMILLAN
EDUCATION

First published 1988

Published by
MACMILLAN EDUCATION LTD
Houndmills, Basingstoke, Hampshire RG21 2XS
and London
Companies and representatives
throughout the world

Typesetting by Footnote Graphics,
Warminster, Wilts.

Printed in Great Britain by
Richard Clay Ltd, Bungay, Suffolk

British Library Cataloguing in Publication Data
Baker, Jill
What next? : post-basic opportunities for
nurses.
1. Great Britain. Medicine. Nursing —
Career guides
I. Title
610.73′023′41
ISBN 0–333–44784–0

Contents

Apologia and Acknowledgements

Throughout this book I have referred to nurses as 'she'. This is simply to avoid the use of 'he and she', 'his and her' and similar expressions, and it is in no way intended to insult the many caring men in the profession. I hope that they will forgive me.

I gratefully acknowledge Mary Waltham for her unfailing encouragement, and Pat Stillwell and Kathy Smithers for their practical help without which this book would have never been written.

Abbreviations Used in the Text

AIDS	Acquired Immune Deficiency Syndrome
BA	Bachelor of Arts
BN	Bachelor of Nursing
BSc	Bachelor of Science
CPN	Community Psychiatric Nurse
CSE	Certificate of Secondary Education
DENCert	District Enrolled Nurse Certificate
DHSS	Department of Health and Social Security
DLC	Distance Learning Centre
DNCert	District Nursing Certificate
EN	Enrolled Nurse
ENB	English National Board for Nursing, Midwifery and Health Visiting
GCE	General Certificate of Education
GCSE	General Certificate of Secondary Education
GP	General Practitioner
MA	Master of Arts
MPhil	Master of Philosophy
MSc	Master of Science
NHS	National Health Service
OHNC	Occupational Health Nursing Certificate
OND	Ophthalmic Nursing Diploma
PCAS	Polytechnic Central Admissions System
PhD	Doctor of Philosophy
RCN	Royal College of Nursing
RGN	Registered General Nurse
RHV	Registered Health Visitor
RM	Registered Midwife
RMN	Registered Mental Nurse
RNMH	Registered Nurse for the Mentally Handicapped
RNT	Registered Nurse Tutor
UCCA	Universities' Central Council on Admissions
UKCC	United Kingdom Central Council for Nursing, Midwifery and Health Visiting

Foreword

In an age where there is an ever-increasing demand for efficient, effective use of resources and public accountability, the need for nurses to plan their career development has never been more urgent. Gone are the days when a basic training sufficed to see the kindly carer through the rest of his or her working life. There is an explosion of new information which is growing all the time, and in order to be able to offer patients the service which they deserve, nurses have to be aware of new developments and continue to learn throughout their professional careers. This is no more than one would expect of any person working in a service-related discipline, but especially important when the 'product' of the service is another human being who has a right to know that the care that is offered is based on sound, up-to-date understanding.

Partly because of the diversity of choices which are open to nurses once they have undertaken their basic preparation, it is not always easy to know which options are available, or the implications of choosing a particular career path. A text such as this, which collates information about these choices, can be a valuable resource when important decisions are made about where to go next. Not only is information provided about formal access to courses, but also something about the work itself and the implications of moving into a particular sphere of nursing.

While information has been collected here about the more formal aspects of career development, it is worth remembering that learning is not confined to the addition of formal qualifications to one's repertoire. One of the important characteristics of all professional people is that they have a curiosity about their work and continue to question and, at times, challenge current practice through self-directed enquiry. Such a characteristic does not have to be confined within the boundaries of a formal course but is an activity which should invade practice at all times.

A combination of both formal and informal enquiry is widely

supported at both national and local levels as evidenced by the recent DHSS video *A Way of Thinking* and its accompanying text. It is recognised that the decisions which nurses have to make about their future careers are not easy, but a wise choice can lead to a rewarding future.

Barbie Vaughan
Senior Tutor
Clinical Practice Development Team
John Radcliffe Hospital School of Nursing
Oxfordshire Health Authority

CHAPTER 1

Introduction

Long gone are the days when the achievement of a basic nursing qualification was an end in itself. Now it is simply the first step on a career path which can lead upwards or sideways in many different directions.

It is the start of many more years of learning, in a formal or informal setting, within a teaching institution or self-directed at home, full time, part time or in your spare time.

What is certain is that, as the profession gathers status and momentum, as we move towards a future in which nursing will be research based and for which the basic training may be seated in higher education, any nurse who wishes to remain caring and competent, let alone progress in her career, will have to take on board the necessity of keeping up to date with developments in her chosen area and broader nursing issues as a whole—and they are likely to increase with the increasing professionalisation of nursing.

What this means in practice is that nurses starting on their professional careers will have to be prepared for a future in which continuing education will play an important part.

This book is intended to guide you through the maze of post-basic education opportunities to suggest how you might begin to plan your future in nursing.

A list of organisations which you might approach for more specialist help is included at the end of this book.

One of the problems which faces everyone emerging from an intensive learning experience, be they nurses or engineers, is that it is hard for them to see further ahead in their lives than the immediate necessity of getting a proper job with some individual status and responsibility and for which they receive the appropriate reward. Of course, post-qualification experience is an important part of any package of skills which you may want to amass to lead you to your next career step, but it is never too early to start to plan your future; even if you change your mind later, skills acquired while moving towards your original aim will not be wasted.

Attendance at study days and seminars which may be of no immediately apparent practical application all help to open your mind to new ideas, to keep it active and alert and to introduce you to new and original thoughts and potentially helpful people. Moreover, attendance at such meetings looks good on your curriculum vitae when you eventually decide to move on.

Even if your ambition takes you no further than wishing to remain at the bedside for the whole of your professional career, your ability to care for your patients will rapidly deteriorate if new concepts and standards are introduced which you do not understand.

Job satisfaction means knowledge of a job well done which is not necessarily acknowledged by others but recognised by yourself, and to achieve this it is important to take every advantage to absorb new ideas, to question and contradict them perhaps, but at least to know of their existence.

The profession and the patients need every single one of such aware nurses. A sensibly planned career may help you to be one.

CHAPTER 2

Planning Your Career

Nursing is probably unique in the enormously varied range of specialisations open to the qualified practitioner. Just because there is such a choice of options, it is very hard sometimes to decide in which direction to go.

If you have no clear idea of the path you want to pursue, then probably the best starting point is yourself.

Realistic self-assessment

In the long run, the success or failure of your choice of career in nursing can depend only on you. Obviously, outside factors have an influence on your happiness and success in any job, but to a very great extent the effect of such factors depends on your reaction to them, on how you are able to face up to problems of various kinds, to deal with them, to solve them or perhaps to be beaten by them.

So first of all, in any career plan, you have to understand yourself in order to choose an avenue which will suit you, your abilities and your temperament.

You probably think you know yourself quite well already. Nonetheless, it is helpful to have things written down, so that you can collate them and absorb them; so I suggest you take the time to consider your own personality and make a few lists about yourself.

These exercises are more usefully undertaken with the help of a friend whose judgement you trust—a friend who will act as enemy. Bear in mind, however, that you are asking your friend to be truthful even if the truth may be unwelcome—don't be insulted when she (or he) is honest about your faults.

What you and your friend together are trying to do is to form a word picture of you, which a third person might use to describe you.

The first list is of, say, ten words which describe your own outstanding characteristics. To help you, I suggest some in Table 2.1. These adjectives are intended to describe you as a person rather than you as a nurse. If, for example, you are basically shy, though you find it easier to communicate when wearing your uniform, then your characteristic is still shy—the uniform is a prop which you use to help to overcome the shyness.

The second list is of your strengths and weaknesses—activities which you undertake day by day and which you may perform competently or with reluctance. Once again, I have made some suggestions in Table 2.2. You may be able to think of others.

If you have persuaded a friend to help you, then you should ask him or her to list your ten outstanding characteristics, and

Table 2.1
Words to describe you as a person

Active	Inquisitive
Adaptable	Intelligent
Aggressive	Meticulous
Ambitious	Panicky
Articulate	Outgoing
Assertive	Passive
Authoritative	Patient
Bossy	Plodding
Brave	Quick-thinking
Careless	Reliable
Cheerful	Reserved
Communicative	Resourceful
Easy-going	Shy
Flexible	Self-confident
Forthright	Self-reliant
Friendly	Studious
Hard-working	Tactful
Impatient	Touchy
Independent	Uncompromising

Table 2.2
Words to describe activities at which you may be good or bad

Advising	Motivating
Asserting yourself	Organising
Budgeting	Persuading
Coping with crises	Planning
Counselling	Remembering
Decision making	Responding to others
Delegating	Taking responsibility
Evaluating	Talking
Explaining	Teaching
Initiating	Timekeeping
Learning	Understanding
Listening	Writing
Making new contacts	

then your particular strengths and weaknesses. Only after you have both made your lists should you compare notes.

It is worth emphasising how important it is for you and your helper to be absolutely honest—and this works in two directions. You must not hesitate to list your own weaknesses; this is not, after all, a job reference and no one apart from you and your trustworthy friend is going to see it. Nor must you be over-modest in listing your strengths. It is only when you have a clear idea of what you can do that you can make an informed decision about what you aspire to be.

The chances are that you and your friend will have put down similar adjectives to describe your characteristics—a good friend will know quite well that you are shy, even if you make enormous efforts to hide it. You may be surprised, however, at the discrepancies in the strengths and weaknesses lists. Quite often, we fail to realise that we are good (or bad) at a particular activity. If you do find discrepancies, then provided that you are certain that your friend is not flattering you (perhaps misleading would be a better word, for she is doing you no favours), you should be guided by your friend's opinion.

If, for example, she believes you are good at coping in crises, then, however panicky you may feel, you are clearly able to hide it and to behave calmly and responsibly, which is what matters.

Table 2.3
Likes and dislikes in nursing

Being in charge	Job security
Being told what to do	Organising the ward
Contact with other health professionals	Pay
	Planning care
Contact with patients	Research
Contact with relatives	Seeing different people week by week
Delivering care	
Hours	Teaching self-care
Institutionalisation	

If she believes you are bad at explaining things to others, she is probably right. Not all of us have the ability to translate what is obvious to us into words that will make it obvious to others.

The final list is one you should make for yourself. It is to set down what you most like and dislike about nursing. Once again I have offered a few suggestions for things to think about (Table 2.3) but I make no judgements about whether they should appear on the credit or debit side of your list. Where you choose to put them—and other things you may think of yourself—will all add to the clues as to which direction you should take.

Now that you have all your lists in front of you, a clearer picture of you should begin to emerge: you as an introvert or an extrovert; you as a doer or a thinker; you as independent or reactive; you as a teacher or a learner; and so on.

Naturally, all this is not definitive, but it will help you as you read through this book to understand which of your particular personal characteristics will enable you to fit into a particular career path and to make a success of it, both for yourself and for those with whom you come into contact. If you choose a specialty for which your own personality is unsuited, the resulting continuing battle with yourself will make you both unhappy and inefficient.

Planning ahead

Next you should examine your own personal circumstances, as these will inevitably have some effect on what you decide to do.

Naturally none of us can be certain what the years ahead will bring, but it is sensible to consider what is likely – or just possible.

What, then, are your commitments? If you are single, heart whole and family free, then you are in the happy position of being able to do more or less as you wish.

Many of you, however, are tied to other people by bonds of love, friendship and duty, and you must be aware when you plan your career of the effect on them. Indeed it may be *for* them as well as yourself that you are setting off hopefully on a path which will lead, if not to fame and fortune, at least to a comfortable and satisfying lifestyle.

No commitment should stop you investigating and then perhaps pursuing the career path you think best, or drive you on along a path you feel is wrong for you. However, I do believe you should understand as best you can what problems you may have to face now and in the future.

Jobs in upper management, for example, require of you long hours and often much travelling – how will your family cope if you are often away from home? Will the high salary compensate for your absence? How will your spouse take to your entering full-time education again? People often feel threatened by partners who are apparently growing up and away into higher intellectual spheres.

Can you afford to keep your family on the salary you will earn as a district nurse? Will you need to move house or to have prior claim to the car? Are your childcare arrangements adequate? Is your mother-in-law likely to have to come to live with you, needing your study as a bedroom?

All these and other difficulties can be met and probably dealt with, but it is only sensible to be aware of them in advance so that you can be ready to cope when you have to.

I am not particularly an advocate of putting things off indefinitely 'until the children are older', 'until my partner gets a promotion' or 'until my lover decides to settle down' – procrastination has a way of turning some time into never with resultant regret and sometimes resentment.

Nevertheless, it may be expedient to delay taking the next step on your career path for a certain period. If this is so, I do urge you to make good use of the intervening time.

If, for example, you are waiting to take up a college place or gaining necessary experience on the wards before setting your sights on promotion, or housekeeping until your children can be cared for by others, do use that time wisely to extend your overall knowledge of the principles and practice of your profession.

Read—certainly the nursing journals but books too, and not only those directly related to the course you intend to pursue. Now is a golden opportunity to enlarge your vision of nursing by extending your reading material to encompass areas new to you; you may not agree with others' views on the philosophy, the policies or the politics of nursing, but you can only gain by knowing they exist and by sharpening your brain in considering why you find them right or wrong.

Have you perhaps time to undertake a course of open learning? Various short- and long-term courses are available to individual nurses which they can follow in their own time and to a certain extent at their own pace. Chapter 11 gives further information on this valuable course of action.

Moreover, this preparation will help you when you finally decide to apply for any formal course of further training. Those deciding who is suitable to take up such training will be looking for evidence of ability, of course, but also for evidence of interest, of self-motivation and of willingness to put effort into and to gain from formalised learning. If in your first letter of application, and later in your interview, you show that you have spent time and effort to inform yourself, then you are well on the way to achieving your training place.

Of course, the same is true for those who seek promotion. If you can show that you have troubled to attend courses or can discuss a recent controversial book or policy at an interview, then you will impress those responsible for the appointment as a serious and worthwhile applicant.

A successful career in nursing, as in any other profession, requires considerable preliminary effort from you before the rewards begin to be apparent.

Once you have decided what your next move is to be, you must start to make the necessary preparations.

Which is the nearest training establishment for you? How will you find the funds? What is the attitude of your own health authority or will you need to apply to another for payment while training?

At the end of this book, I have listed useful addresses and sources of information, and now is the time to send off letters or to make telephone calls. Much information is available, both from nursing organisations and from the training establishments themselves, but you will have to ask for it.

Moreover, staff already working in the area in which you are interested will prove a rich source of help if you ask them. If it seems appropriate, do not neglect to enlist the help of your health authority's nurse tutor in charge of post-basic training (if you have one). Find out by ringing up the school of nursing and asking, 'Could you tell me the name of the tutor in charge of post-basic training? I should like to write to her.' You do not have to reveal your own name.

Once you have gathered together all these details and have decided exactly what you want to do, then you are ready to start to do it.

Bear in mind that applications for course places are often required months or (with some very popular specialties) even a year or so in advance of the start of the course; so do not leave everything to the last minute.

Now, with the details of the course and yourself gathered around you and your mind quite clear as to why you want to take it, you can start to apply.

How to apply

First of all, let me give you a word of warning. Some of what I have to say in this section may be difficult for some of you to accept. My advice may go against your natural inclinations to such an extent that you feel unable to take it. However, this section is written assuming that you want to be accepted for the course or job you apply for; what I am doing here is to suggest how you are most likely to succeed, taking into account that those responsible for choosing candidates are looking for particular personal characteristics as well as evidence of intellectual ability.

9

Your object is to sell yourself as the best person for the course or job, and there are at least some measures you can take which will afford you a good start towards this end.

Letters of application

Whatever your next career step is to be, you will need to write a letter of application—for a course place, for a job at a higher grade, and so on. I cannot, I think, overestimate the importance of this first letter, particularly if there is likely to be stiff competition for whatever you are after.

Your letter is the first intimation to those responsible for the appointment that you exist, and it *must* convey the impression of a serious nurse who is capable, intelligent and thoughtful. In other words, your letter of application is selling you to a buyer who has yet to be convinced that she wants you.

It is worth spending some time on your letter, preparing a first draft, reading and correcting it before you make a final copy.

What follows is a list of 'dos' and 'don'ts'. I apologise if they seem obvious to some of you. If they were obvious to everyone, I need not have put this section in at all but apparently they are not clearly evident to all.

- **Do** take the time and trouble to make your letter look efficient and capable. If you make a mistake, start again on a fresh piece of paper.

- **Do** include a sentence or two explaining your qualifications, even if they are also included in your curriculum vitae or application form.

- **Do** type or write neatly in blue or black ink, and not in pencil or an odd colour, and use the same pen throughout.

- **Do** enclose a stamped addressed envelope to encourage a reply. (Even a prompt 'No' is better than no answer at all—and most organisations are sometimes guilty of neglecting to answer applicants.)

10

- **Do** ensure that there are no spelling or grammatical mistakes in your letter. (If you cannot spell, use a dictionary. If your grammar is shaky, use short sentences. Get a friend to check your draft if you think it wise.)

- **Don't** write on hospital writing paper. (An application is personal, and to use institutional writing paper is stealing, if in a mild way.)

- **Don't** write on coloured, fancy or (what is worse) scented writing paper. (An application is a serious matter and requires a different approach from a letter to a friend.)

- **Don't** write on a scruffy piece of lined paper torn out of your notebook. (An application should look as if you have given it serious thought and not scribbled hurriedly in your tea break.)

- **Don't** get the name of the person or the institution to which you are applying wrong. (To do so is evidence of carelessness—not the impression you are trying to convey—and, moreover, it is rude.)

- **Don't** address the person to whom you are applying by her first name unless you know her very well indeed. (It is difficult to offend by being too formal, but it is easy to offend by being too informal. If the name of the person to whom you are to apply does not indicate a title (that is, applications to Jill Baker), then Miss or Ms Baker are both acceptable.)

Your letter of application should look similar to the following.

27 Grafton Gardens
Lindsell
Essex EX1 3GP

2 September 1988

Miss J. Johnson
Department of Community Studies
Lindsell College of Further Education
Lindsell
Essex EX1 2PG

Dear Miss Johnson,

I should like to be considered for a place on the Lindsell College health visiting course starting in September 1989. I am a registered nurse and have recently completed my midwifery training in preparation for undertaking health visitor training. I have also attended a short course on child nutrition organised by my health authority.

I enclose my curriculum vitae together with a stamped addressed envelope.

I look forward to hearing from you.

Yours sincerely,

Clare Green.

CLARE GREEN

Although many health authorities and educational establishments supply application forms for candidates to complete, on other occasions your letter of application will need to be accompanied by a curriculum vitae—a table of information about yourself and your achievements to date.

It is in any event a good idea to prepare one for yourself and to keep it on file, updating it as the occasion demands. Without it, you may find that you have forgotten just when you completed a particular course or took up an earlier post to which you may wish to refer later.

It is quite a useful memorandum to have with you when you go for an interview, so that you can be sure that what you put on the application form tallies with what you are telling the interviewer.

Your curriculum vitae should be neatly prepared and succinct. Interviewers do not want your autobiography—despite what those whose job it is to prepare curricula vitae for cash may tell you. Interviewers want a clear easy-to-read list of your personal details, qualifications and previous posts. Other useful information can be appended, but not, please, a subjective list of your qualities, as in the current American idiom; they will prefer to ferret out these for themselves.

Your curriculum vitae should be similar to the following. The last comment about the referees is, of course, optional.

As you will see I have included the headings **Sex** and **Marital status** on my curriculum vitae form and you may find similar questions on an application form. You may believe that neither of these is relevant or the concern of anyone other than yourself. However, it is normal still to include them, and that brings me to the possibly unacceptable advice I mentioned earlier in this section.

It is my view that it is unwise in letters of application (and in interviews) to draw particular attention to views or attitudes you hold which may not be universally accepted. Clearly, it would be wrong to misrepresent your views if you are directly questioned, but it is not in your own best interests to overemphasise opinions to which the person reading the form may not be sympathetic.

Curriculum vitae

Name:

Address:

Telephone number:

Date of birth:

Sex:

Marital status:

Qualifications:
　O and A levels:
　Nursing qualifications:
　Other qualifications:

Posts held (in date order):

Other relevant information:

Referees:
(A)
(B)

Optional (Please do not approach Miss A or Mrs B without letting me know.)

There are two reasons for this. The first is simply that those responsible for appointments, like the rest of us, have prejudices of their own which, if they conflict strongly with yours, may influence the outcome of your application. (You may simply not get an interview if you announce your opinions in a letter.) However, less cynically and more importantly, an interviewer may feel that overemphasis of a point of view not widely acceptable to the general public is an inappropriate attitude in someone aspiring to a course or job which brings them into contact with a wide variety of people. In other words, it is not your opinion which will lose you the place on the course or the job, but your unsound judgement in pushing it forward in an inappropriate setting.

So, if you are gay or a member of an extreme political party or an ardent feminist, try not to let your views colour your application, even if only to the extent of leaving blank lines on the form or omitting usual information from your curriculum vitae. Fill in all the information you are required to give, if you can bring yourself to do so.

If you feel very strongly, then leave the lines blank, but remember you have chosen to do so; it is then the prerogative of the person reading the form to draw what conclusions she wishes from your omissions. And people, rightly or wrongly, do make those sorts of judgement.

It is relevant here to mention your choice of referees. These should be people who can testify to your professional ability — and chosen from a rank higher than you. If possible, they should be from different arenas: a tutor from your school of nursing and a senior nurse, for example. It is usual to nominate two of them, and it is impolite to do so without telling them. However, if you cannot tell them because you are unwilling yet to announce your intention of moving on, then this is not a disaster. It is unusual to take up references until the end of the application process and you may get the chance to warn them later on. If you think that there is a chance that someone will be offended by being asked for a reference for you without prior warning, don't nominate her in the first place. It is perfectly acceptable to request that referees are not approached without telling you — you can include such a request on your curriculum vitae or application form.

Interview technique

In order to obtain a course place—and of course to gain promotion—you will be required to undergo one or more face-to-face interviews. Such interviews are testing occasions even for the very self-confident; for most of us, they are agonising. Here I offer some suggestions on how to face an interview, which I hope will help you give of your best.

First of all, whether your interview is to be with one person or a group, it is important that you should feel as relaxed as possible in such testing circumstances. I suggest therefore that it is essential policy on your part to have prepared yourself well before the day.

Sometimes you will be offered the opportunity of an informal visit before the actual interview day. Take it if you possibly can. You will be able to size up the institution and to discover whether you would be happy there. Moreover, you can, during the visit, ask questions which would not be appropriate at a formal interview and take mental notes about points on which you could sensibly ask for further information at interview.

If you do not have the chance of an informal visit before the interview, find out in advance how to reach the address to which you have been summoned and how long it will take you to get there. Decide what you will wear and make sure it is ready. Gather together in advance any documents you need to take with you including your curriculum vitae or a copy of your application form. Think up some questions to ask concerning the content of the course or its administration or, if you are going to a job interview, about opportunities for professional development. Any questions of a professional nature will do, so long as they are not inane; their purpose is to make you seem to be taking an intelligent and informed interest.

On the day, set off in plenty of time. Interviewers are busy people and may not take kindly to being kept waiting; to be late may fluster you and imply to them a lack of serious intent.

If by a horrible mischance you are going to be late, telephone to say so, and to request a change of time. Do not simply appear long after your appointment time and expect to be seen. If you are very early, either go for a short walk or sit quietly in the waiting room. Do not be tempted to pop into Sainsbury's; you will either spend more time than you intended or burden yourself with scruffy carriers.

Now, a word about clothing—as I said before, the interview is not an appropriate time to make a controversial statement either by your dress or by your demeanour. You can do all that later once you have been accepted for what you want. Now is the time to try to match up to what your interviewer will probably hope to see: a candidate who is not so extreme in any way that she risks offending the interviewer now or—more importantly—the patients or clients later. Leave at home the badges proclaiming your sexual or political orientation. They are irrelevant and as inappropriate for an interview as they are in the homes or by the bedside of patients who may mistrust your nursing skills as a result of them.

If you must make a statement, then that of course is your right; it is the right of the interviewer to conclude that your demeanour is inappropriate in one aspiring to be a teacher or whatever. Once again it is not the views themselves that are being judged; rather judgement is being passed on your decision to flaunt your views where they may offend.

On time and looking unexceptional, you reach the interview room. Ideally an interview should be a two-way conversation, and a skilled interviewer will phrase the questions in such a way that you are unable to answer them with a straight 'Yes' or 'No'. However, even if the interviewer is not so skilled, do try to enlarge on your answers a little, for example

Interviewer: 'I see you took the RMN course in Oxford.'
You: 'Yes. It was fascinating to be in a university city, even though not part of the university itself. There really was an atmosphere of learning, and I felt that helped me.'

The addition of the enlargement enables the interviewer to take you on from there.

You are trying to establish some rapport with your interviewer, and you can only do this if the conversation flows fairly freely. This is why I suggest you arm yourself with one or two questions beforehand; if there is an awkward gap, you can fill it with a question.

Some interviewers have been on courses where they have learnt to use the direct personal question to disconcert you. You should be prepared for this.

A currently popular pair of questions is

'What do you think you are good (best) at?'

which is followed closely by 'And what are you bad (worst) at?'

Answer promptly and truthfully if you can, while not of course dwelling on your faults. The lists you made earlier will help you, and it is sensible when admitting to a weakness or gap in experience to add that you are trying to amend it in some way. Don't bridle or giggle.

If you feel that a question is an intrusion on your personal life, try to say so firmly but without anger or whining and try not to harangue the interviewer. It is possible, though difficult, to extricate yourself from such an exchange, leaving the interviewer with a greater respect for you as a confident and reasonable adult—perhaps something along these lines:

Interviewer: 'Are you gay?'

You: 'I'm disappointed that you felt it necessary to ask me that. It doesn't seem to me to be relevant, though if it is, perhaps you could explain why.'

It may help you to respond more easily to personal questions if you understand that the interviewer, when seeing candidates, has to bear in mind not only you but also her colleagues, the established team and the patients, and is trying to select someone who will work well within an existing framework with its own group dynamics. She would be unwise, for example, to let down her team by appointing someone who is likely to be a frequent absentee and that is why she asks searching questions about your child care arrangements. Answer as politely as you can; once you have got the job, you will be in a stronger position to start agitating for a crèche.

Try hard to keep calm but, if you do finally become angry, don't be too upset about it later. You would have been unhappy working in that environment anyway.

Above all, don't be tempted to tell lies or mislead at interviews. Skilled interviewers may suspect; they have seen similar situations before, and you run the risk that your lie will be discovered later when you have more to lose.

Towards the end of the interview, it is likely that you will be asked whether you have questions. Here is where those you have prepared beforehand are useful, if you have not already used them. Try to make your first questions at least orientated towards professional issues rather than personal questions. In other words, it is better to say

'Could you expand a little on what teaching practice entails?'

rather than

'How much holiday do I get?'

Most interviewers are kindly disposed towards those they interview and will try to help you to help yourself to appear in a good light. They have been on the receiving end themselves, and it is after all in their own best interests to get an accurate view of the candidate's potential. It is not usually until you reach the higher echelons of management that really tough interviewing techniques turn up. Then it is not unusual for the interviewer to be deliberately provocative, in order to see how candidates react under stress.

However, if you do have the misfortune to come across an interviewer having a bad day, do try to keep calm and to answer unreasonable questions reasonably. Don't lose your temper. Remember that unpleasantness to which you are being sub-jected may be simply a ploy and, if you respond well, you will gain high marks.

If the interviewer is utterly high-handed and overbearing, defuse your temper by recognising that she is merely revealing her own incompetence at interviewing and probably is secretly aware that she is not good at the job. If she is truly nasty, then maybe you do not want to work under or learn from her anyway. You too are entitled to a choice.

Good luck with your interviews. Don't let one failure put you off. Try again . . . and again. Someone out there wants each one of us. It may take you a little time to discover who that someone is, but one of the secrets of success is a confident manner. If you believe in yourself, others will believe in you too.

CHAPTER 3

Project 2000

As this book goes to press, the recommendations of the UKCC's report *Project 2000 — A New Preparation for Practice* (published in May 1986) are still under discussion. However, as they propose radical changes in the way nurse education is delivered, it is vital for nurses—and particularly those at the beginning of their careers—to be aware of them. Project 2000 is likely to affect everyone nursing to some extent and may eventually make a profound difference to your career.

Basically, the original proposals were that all nurse learners should share a common foundation programme (for a period of time yet to be decided, but up to 2 years) and then follow a branch programme in mental illness, mental handicap, nursing of adults or nursing of children (for a period of time which completes a 3-year learning programme). This would lead to registration as a nurse practitioner with the UKCC.

Project 2000 went on to recommend that specialist practitioners be identified in all areas of practice, and listed health visiting, occupational health nursing, school nursing, district nursing, community psychiatric nursing and community mental handicap nursing as specialist qualifications for the community.

Moreover, after registration a coherent framework of continuing education should be developed for all registered practitioners.

Perhaps the key recommendations in Project 2000 were that student nurses should be supernumerary to NHS staffing establishments and that they should receive training grants, rather than salaries, though still primarily controlled by the NHS and administered from a separate education budget.

This would of course bring student nurses into line with

students in other disciplines, and the report went on to suggest that links with other educational establishments be pursued, together with joint academic and professional validation of qualifications.

The report also recommended the improvement of the position of teaching staff and the enhancement of their own opportunities for further education. Teaching qualifications at degree level should be established for teachers of nursing, midwifery and health visiting.

Moreover, those whose teaching takes place 'on the job' rather than in the classroom should have formal preparation for this role.

Finally, Project 2000 recommended the end of enrolled nurse training, the enhancement of opportunities for enrolled nurses already on the register to convert to RGNs, RMNs, RNMHs or RSCNs and the establishment of an entirely new grade of 'helper' to be directly supervised by a registered practitioner.

A new organisational structure should be created to implement these proposals.

A full list of the original 25 Project 2000 proposals will be found at the end of this chapter.

After the publication of Project 2000, a period of about 5 months was allowed for comment from the profession. Meetings were held nationwide and debate was full and wide ranging. Over 2500 submissions from organisations and individuals were received: about 1900 from individuals, 600 from informal groups and 40 from formal organisations.

Most of the submissions were in broad agreement with the aim of Project 2000 to change and improve the education of nurses.

However, many important modifications were suggested and in some particular areas—notably midwifery, mental handicap and mental illness nursing—deep concern was expressed that the special skills necessary would become submerged within the greater ocean of general nursing.

The new role of the 'helper' raised many fears as did the future of the enrolled nurse.

Doubts were expressed by almost all who commented on the report about the availability of enough money from government and manpower within the profession to institute such radical changes without cutting corners—or indeed even to begin to institute the changes.

Nevertheless, there was wide acceptance of the principles of the report and that was sufficient for it to progress to the next stage.

When the submissions had been coordinated and considered, a final version of the report was finally sent early in 1987 to the Secretary of State for Health, then Norman Fowler, for his consideration.

In April and May 1987 the run-up to the general election brought commitment to Project 2000 implementation from the Alliance, but the other parties were more circumspect. In the event, the Conservatives were returned to power and a new Secretary of State for Health, John Moore, appointed.

By this time, Project 2000 had been sent for comment to the health authorities in the UK with a deadline for comment of August 1987.

But still, as this book goes to press, we await a statement from Health Secretary John Moore on the Government's acceptance or otherwise of the Project 2000 proposals and the financial allocation necessary to implement them.

The nursing establishment is fully committed to Project 2000. Indeed, without it, the future of nursing is bleak. Already innovators in nursing education are piloting basic training schemes which incorporate many features of the proposals. Such schemes link schools of nursing with other educational establishments, and incorporate new teaching and learning methods, and changes in curriculum content and design.

Action is urgently needed to try to halt the dramatic fall in the numbers of nurses entering basic training which is having a knock-on effect on post-basic education. For as health authorities concentrate available cash on their own immediate recruitment needs, they are tending to neglect post-basic education.

Indeed, the ENB has made a separate bid to take over the funding of continuing and post-basic education, in the belief that a central funding programme would allow concentration of effort where the need is greatest. For, despite increasing emphasis on community care, the number of nurses seconded to health-visitor and district-nurse training has fallen in the past 10 years. And the shortage of nurses trained in particular clinical specialties has become a national concern.

Meanwhile the Board plans to improve its overworked career advice service by increasing staffing levels and by computerising information on available courses.

But all this is for the future.

Clearly, many months and years of groundwork are going to be needed—and pilot projects set up and evaluated—before the finally agreed recommendations of Project 2000 can be implemented on anything like a national scale.

This book assumes the pre-Project 2000 *status quo* as far as post-basic training is concerned. Nevertheless, anyone who has career prospects in view in the short or long term would be well advised to watch Project 2000 and ENB developments, as they may well have a bearing on how your future education will be conducted—and on how you need to prepare yourself for it. Nursing is clearly moving towards a sounder academic base and nothing you do now to improve your own academic standing can possibly be wasted.

The original proposals

The following 25 proposals formed the core of the Project 2000 report. Whether and how they will be implemented remains to be seen. Nonetheless it is important to be aware of them, and to take them into account as a pointer towards future developments when considering your future nursing career.

1. There should be a new registered practitioner competent to assess the need for care, to provide care, to monitor and evaluate, and to do this in institutional and non-institutional settings.
2. Preparation for the new registered practitioner should normally be completed within 3 years.
3. All preparation for registration should begin with a common foundation programme followed by branch programmes.
4. The common foundation programme should be a substantial part of preparation, lasting up to 2 years.
5. Branch programmes should be available in mental illness, mental handicap, nursing of adults and nursing of children, with experimentation in a branch for midwifery.

24

6. In the case of midwifery, there should also be an 18-month post-registration preparation.
7. There should be a new single list of competencies applicable to all registered practitioners at the level of registration and set out in training rules.
8. All future practitioners should register with the UKCC. The area of practice should be indicated on the register.
9. Midwives should debate the new registered practitioner outcomes in the light of their special needs.
10. There should be a coherent comprehensive cost-effective framework of education beyond registration.
11. There should be specialist practitioners, some of whom will also be team leaders, in all areas of practice in hospital and community settings. The requisite specialist qualifications will be recordable on the UKCC's register.
12. Health visiting, occupational health and school nursing should be specialist qualifications in health promotion which are recordable on the UKCC's register.
13. District nursing, community psychiatric nursing and community mental handicap nursing should be specialist qualifications which are recordable on the UKCC's register.
14. Students should be supernumerary to NHS staffing establishments throughout the whole period of preparation.
15. There should be a new helper, directly supervised and monitored by a registered practitioner.
16. Students should receive training grants which are primarily NHS controlled. These should be administered via the national boards and should derive from a separately identified education budget.
17. The position of teaching staff should be improved with a view to enhancing performance and allowing teachers opportunities for further training and for full participation in wider educational activities.
18. The full range of means to achieve the appropriate concentrations of educational resources should be considered, including re-establishments, partnerships, consortia, etc.
19. Educational costs should be clearly identified and heads of educational institutions should be given responsibility for

management of a more comprehensive and clearly de-
lineated education budget.
20. Practitioners should have formal preparation for teaching
    roles in practice settings.
21. Moves should be made to establish teaching qualifications at
    degree level for teachers of nursing, midwifery and health
    visiting.
22. Joint professional and academic validation should be
    pursued from the very outset of change in order to achieve
    academic recognition for professional qualifications.
23. Programmes of training for entry for the enrolled nurse part
    of the register should cease as soon as is practicable.
24. The enhancement of opportunities for enrolled nurses to
    enter RGN, RMN, RNMH and RSCN parts of the register
    should now be given priority.
25. Urgent consideration should be given to creating a new
    organisational structure to implement the proposals of
    Project 2000.

CHAPTER 4

Further Statutory Training

A number of nurses who have completed their basic training for one part of the register—RGNs, RSCNs, RMNs, or RNMHs—go on at some time to a further course of basic training for another part. Thus, we find RGNs who are also RMNs, RNMHs who go on to register as RGNs, and so on.

There are a number of reasons for this—not least of which is the view that a general nursing qualification, in addition to another basic nursing qualification, stands the holder in better stead for promotion to management posts in the future.

However, for many nurses the reason for undertaking a second basic training is that, during their general training, they have had a taste of another specialty which they then decide to pursue further, either immediately or after a few years, simply for their own interest and satisfaction in that area of care.

Whatever the reason, once you have achieved the first basic qualification, a course of training for another part of the register is much shorter than that undertaken by a new student (Table 4.1). The fact that the lengths of time differ indicates the extent to which the syllabuses for the different specialties overlap.

Obviously, training courses for general nurses and sick children's nurses have in common a concentration on physical disease, anatomy and physiology and have traditionally concentrated on institutional care and how to deliver it. Newer programmes, however, are endeavouring to direct the emphasis of care away from a predominantly institutional model. The training for mental illness and mental handicap nurses, certainly, concentrates more on sociology, psychology and psychiatry, on responsibility, taking and giving, to an extent on care in the institutional setting, but increasingly on community-

Table 4.1
Typical training times for registered nurses to achieve entry to another part of the register

What you want to train for

	RGN	RSCN	RMN	RNMH
RGN	—	13 months	18 months	18 months
RSCN	18 months	—	18 months	18 months
RMN	18 months	18 months	—	12 months
RNMH	18 months	18 months	12 months	—

What you are already

based care and its management. Nurses considering undertaking a second statutory training may find much that is very different and new in their second course. It is not a particularly easy option.

Besides your basic qualification, you will have to fulfil the individual entry requirements of the school of nursing you wish to enter; these may be academic (usually five O levels or, for more mature students, a written test of ability) and others (most schools of nursing have an upper age limit, for example).

Courses are held at schools of nursing and you should apply to the director of nurse education at the school you choose. If at first you do not succeed, try again.

You will, of course, revert to student status while you are undertaking a second statutory training and be paid at student rates.

Further information on schools of nursing is available from

the Central Register and Clearing House, or the *Directory of Schools of Nursing*.

Enrolled nurses

At the time of writing this book, there were many enrolled nurses throughout the country desperately chasing the tiny number of places on so-called 'conversion' courses, which enabled them to upgrade from enrolled to registered nurse. As those few places very often went to 'local' enrolled nurses, it was almost impossible to find a place and, meanwhile, funding for such places as there were was drying up.

Aside from training as a district enrolled nurse (Chapter 6), becoming an occupational health nurse, or undertaking one of the specialist clinical courses designed for enrolled nurses (Chapter 7), there is very little currently on offer for the enrolled nurse who wants to enlarge her career horizons. One of the possibilities, oddly enough, is to obtain some A levels and to embark on a mature entrant degree, or to join the Open University. Neither of these is much help towards a straight-forward career in nursing practice but may open new oppor-tunities. Another is to obtain five O levels and to start again from scratch, but this seems a thoroughly backward way of going forward. Midwifery takes three years and five O levels too.

The best hope for the enrolled nurse lies in Project 2000 (see Chapter 3). Its recommendations embodied the 'enhancement' of opportunities for enrolled nurses to upgrade to RGN, RMN, RNMH or RSCN–in other words, to become a registered practitioner. The Royal College of Nursing went further in its evidence on Project 2000 by recommending that all enrolled nurses who elected to do so should be enabled to convert to RGN, while those who did not so choose might remain as they were. One way or another, implementation of the Project 2000 recommendations should bring about some improvement in prospects for enrolled nurses who want to enhance their careers–though the extent of that improvement is undeter-mined and the time scale is not clear.

Meanwhile, however, enrolled nurses are at a disadvantage and no amount of well-meaning empty words will disguise the fact or do anything to help those who want to move on.

CHAPTER 5

Midwifery

The midwife is an independent practitioner in her own right; indeed it is possible to enter midwifery training direct if you have the necessary O levels. However, most midwives have first trained as nurses.

An astonishingly large proportion of those who train as midwives do so not as an end in itself but as part of a planned career progression. A midwifery qualification, for example, is the alternative to an obstetric course which is sometimes hard to obtain as a prerequisite to health visitor training (see Chapter 6). Moreover, those who plan to work abroad often see midwifery as necessary for practice overseas, and there is no doubt that, for those who hope to work in the Third World countries, it is certainly an important attribute.

The result is a continuing shortage of midwives. Yet midwifery is, for those who do practise, a constantly satisfying and rewarding career, and one which offers prospects of increasing clinical expertise, or moves into management, teaching or research.

Much of the midwife's work is with normal healthy mothers and babies—and with the rest of the family too—and her role is one of enabling and supporting rather than 'nursing' in the generally understood sense of the word. That is one reason why many practising midwives are so reluctant to be considered simultaneously with the rest of the nursing profession, instead preferring to emphasise their very different role of caring predominantly for the well.

The midwife is concerned with the health and well-being of mother and baby through pregnancy, birth and the post-partum period. She is trained to deliver babies herself but must have both the knowledge and the responsibility to decide whether medical intervention is necessary.

All this means that one of the most important attributes of a good midwife is an interest in and liking for women – a sentimental fondness for small babies is not enough.

You must be a good listener; many women now have strong views on how the birth of their baby should be conducted and it is up to the midwife to help them to achieve their aims—within the policy of the local health district and the safety of the mother and child. Sometimes the desires of the mother will conflict with those of others concerned with the birth—the GP, the hospital and the midwife herself—and in such cases it is the midwife who will find herself in the centre of controversy. You will have to be sufficiently strong to cope with the demands of all sides while keeping the well-being of mother and child firmly in view.

Moreover, you must be sensitive enough to respond to the unspoken demands of the women under your care. Not everyone is able to voice the special anxieties of pregnancy; the midwife must be alert to recognise the signs and to encourage a need to discuss possible problems with an informed and sympathetic person.

The midwife is also an educator—guiding pregnant women to care for their own health and that of their baby. You must be able to talk sympathetically and persuasively and, while continuing to try, be tolerant towards those who have failed to take your advice.

Tolerance is an important asset to a midwife. If you are inclined to become impatient and exasperated with those whose illness is to some extent self-inflicted, or who make no effort to improve, how are you going to cope with those mothers who are unable or unwilling to make the effort to care for their own health or that of their unborn baby? They are entitled to your best care; will you be able to give it?

Nor are all babies eagerly awaited. As a midwife, you may be caring at the same time for women who are desperately miserable because they are pregnant and others who are desperately miserable because they have miscarried. You will need the maturity to recognise the validity of different circumstances, and the wisdom to modify your approach appropriately.

You must be prepared to work sometimes irregular hours and at night. Babies—and false labours—recognise no clock.

If you are a man planning to train as a midwife—and it is only in this decade that men have been allowed to train in the UK—be prepared to meet some prejudice, both from other members of the profession and from some of your clients, and understand that women from some ethnic groups have religious or social reasons for refusing your services.

Acceptance of male midwives is by no means universal yet.

Nevertheless, there has for the past few years been something of a revolution taking place in midwifery practice. Much-publicised work of such pioneers as Leboyer, a French obstetrician, together with the strong views of many midwives have brought about a change in the attitude of many women.

While women were previously content to allow birth to be managed for them and to submit to medical procedures without questioning, they are now increasingly seeking to control their own bodies and to participate actively in the birth process. They expect the midwife to partner their endeavour.

The extent to which these views are supported and encouraged differs from hospital to hospital, from GP to GP, and from midwifery manager to midwifery manager. Before you embark on midwifery training, it is sensible to consider a little where your own sympathies lie and to discover whether the midwifery unit in which you hope to train practises methods with which you can live.

If your views are radical, I suggest you will be unhappy training within a unit where medical intervention is routine and women's own preferences are dismissed as uninformed and inconvenient.

On the other hand, if you believe that the safest and most sensible way to have a baby is in hospital and that the professionals always know best, then you may equally be unhappy in a unit which leads the field in radical techniques.

Most units try to tread the middle path. Many now agree a 'birth plan' with mothers to be, allowing women to set out their preferences regarding position, pain relief and so on, but with a cautionary 'if possible' attached which allows the midwife to intervene when she feels it important.

A midwife may work in hospital or in the community or—in

some districts—part of the time in hospital and the rest of the time in the community.

The midwife in hospital

In hospital, her areas of concern are the ante-natal clinic, where pregnant women come increasingly often as pregnancy advances for routine physical examination. For some women these visits are the only opportunity they will have for learning about what will happen during the birth of their baby, and it is an important time for the midwife both to offer help and advice and to listen to worries and fears.

Women also come to the clinic for scanning and amniocentesis and the reassurance of the midwife is especially essential during these unfamiliar and perhaps frightening experiences.

During routine clinic visits, the midwife hopes to lay the foundation of a trusting relationship with the women she may later help through the birth and post-partum period. There is, of course, no guarantee that she will be on duty when 'her' mothers give birth.

The midwife may also work in the ante-natal ward where she will be caring for women who have been admitted early because of a potential or actual problem, and here again there will be great emphasis on the emotional care and support the midwife must be able to give, whatever the circumstances of admission.

In the labour ward the midwife will be on hand to support and monitor the mother and baby—and the father or others involved—during the stages of labour. If all goes well, she will conduct the delivery herself and she is trained in the use of pain control techniques and drugs, but it is also her responsibility to recognise the appearance of potential problems and to call for medical assistance when necessary, meanwhile setting emergency procedures in motion. In the post-natal ward, the midwife cares for mother and baby, ensuring that their physical progress is normal. She will help the new mother to establish breast feeding if that is appropriate or will oversee bottle feeding routines. She will teach the new mother how to care for her baby, in the hope that good practice learnt in hospital will be continued when mother and child return home.

Most of the preceding paragraphs refer to normal pregnancy and delivery, but of course not all are. To share the joy of healthy parents delighted with a newly born child is naturally a wonderfully satisfying and elating experience. However, it is an equally important part of the midwife's role to share the grief and to try to bring some comfort to those parents whose baby dies or is born ill or disabled. They may wish to talk or to keep silent and the midwife must be sensitive to and respond to their needs.

Some midwives choose to work in a special care baby unit or intensive care unit where premature or sick babies are cared for in highly controlled conditions. Here, too, besides the well-being of the babies, the emotional needs and concerns of the parents are of great importance and it is the midwife who can decide how they can best be involved in caring for their child.

In the community

The extent of the community midwife's involvement in an individual pregnancy and birth depends very much on the area in which she practises. In some districts all mothers are routinely booked into general hospital beds and visit the hospital clinic for most routine examinations. The community midwife will thus be involved in only some ante-natal and post-natal care and rarely with the birth itself. However, she may conduct or take part in ante-natal classes, talking to groups of mothers (and some fathers) about the progress of pregnancy and childbirth, teaching techniques of relaxation and breathing, and discussing ways of feeding and caring for babies and general parentcraft. She will probably make one ante-natal visit to the mother's home.

She will not see the family again, however, until mother and baby return home from hospital after the birth. Every mother is entitled to a daily visit from a midwife for 10 days following birth, to check that she and the baby are progressing satisfactorily and, if she is discharged from hospital before 10 days are up, then the visits will be made by the community midwife.

Elsewhere, the community midwife may be the mother's chief support, and in this case she may also conduct a home confinement or follow the mother to the GP unit or hospital to oversee the birth there.

Between these two extremes, the amount of inter-personal relationship between midwife and mothers differs in different districts.

Many of those who train as midwives have in view the prospect of working in the community, where there is likely to be a greater opportunity to build up individual relationships and certainly greater responsibility for managing your own case load and practising your skills in the way you prefer. It is worth pointing out, however, that midwives applying for community posts will be expected to have had perhaps 2 years' experience in hospital after qualifying, in order to consolidate their experience and to build up their confidence in their own practice.

Private midwifery

A small but increasing number of midwives practise privately.

Disillusion with the system—a feeling that having a baby in hospital under the NHS is rather like being one of a number of battery chickens, a process which takes account of neither individuality nor personal needs—has produced both midwives who want to care for mothers on a one-to-one basis and mothers who want that too.

For a lump sum, somewhere in the region of £700, a private midwife will attend a mother in her own home as often and for as long as necessary during pregnancy, birth and the post-partum period.

As the midwife is an independent practitioner in her own right, she is entitled to practise in this way but, like any other self-employed person, she loses the security both of a regular income and pension and of group support to a certain extent if she chooses to practise in this way. Moreover, it is likely that her clients will all come from the same stratum of society.

Nevertheless, there is no doubt that demand for private midwifery services is increasing and that job satisfaction is more certain for those who control their own practice.

Qualifications

It is possible to enter midwifery direct, though only very few midwives are trained in this way, currently in just one school, though others are interested, and even a degree course is under consideration. The minimum age for direct entry is 17 years old and you need five O levels including English language and one science subject. Training takes 3 years.

It also takes 3 years of training to qualify as a midwife if you enter having first trained as a nurse in mental illness or mental handicap, as an enrolled nurse or as a sick children's nurse, and you need the same five O levels.

Only if you are a qualified RGN or SRN are you eligible for the shorter 18-month course to become an RM (registered midwife).

You will be employed by the health authority as a student midwife. The first section of your training will be in hospital, where you will spend part of the time in the midwifery school and part of the time in the clinics and wards, learning about the normal physical processes of pregnancy and birth, and its psychological effects on the mother and the rest of the family.

In the next stage of training, the student midwife works in the community alongside an experienced community midwife who has undergone extra training in teaching others.

Finally, she returns to the hospital to consolidate her understanding of normal childbirth and to study ways of pain relief, to learn about abnormalities and complications, to gain some experience of special care baby units, and to study professional and social legislation.

At this stage, the student will be ready to care for mothers, under supervision, during all the stages of childbirth.

The student's work is assessed throughout the course, and at the end she has to undergo both oral and written examinations.

Funding

Student midwives, like student nurses, are employed by the health authority in which their training takes place and are considered to be part of the workforce. If you are accepted for training, you will be paid as any employee. You should apply first to the director of midwifery services at the hospital or unit you have chosen.

A word of warning—it would not be sensible to confess at interview to an intention to undertake midwifery training simply so that you can go on to be a health visitor!

And after that . . .

For many midwives it is enough to continue in practice for the rest of their careers. If this is what you choose to do, you will be required to undertake a refresher course every 5 years to ensure that your practice has kept up with the times and that you are continuing to give the best possible care.

There are, too, short courses relevant to midwifery practice which you can apply to undertake, such as the ENB course on intensive care of the newborn.

You can, if you are practising in the community, undertake training which will allow you to supervise students working in the community. You can go on to the Advanced Diploma in Midwifery or, if you want to teach full time, the Midwife Teacher's Diploma—more about these in Chapter 9.

If your bent is for organisation, midwifery is managed by midwives and you can apply for promotion in the usual way.

Further information

The following national organisations will supply further information, and their addresses will be found at the end of this book:

- Appropriate national board for nursing, midwifery and health visiting.
- UKCC Professional Officer (Midwifery).
- Royal College of Midwives.
- Midwifery Adviser, Royal College of Nursing.
- Your local school of midwifery.
- Association of Radical Midwives.

CHAPTER 6

Nursing in the Community

If you are independent and self-reliant, if you enjoy building up relationships and, above all, if you are adaptable enough to take responsibility yourself and to enable and allow your patients to take it too, then the community may be the place for you.

As a sweeping generalisation, nurses in the community setting provide the nursing interventions appropriate to enable their clients to maintain as nearly as possible a 'normal' healthy lifestyle in their own homes. This means that the nurse sees her patients on their own ground, rather than in the artificial and organised atmosphere of the hospital, and must be prepared to some extent to accept their values rather than to impose her own.

If you are hurt by rejection of your offers of help or impatient with those who do not or cannot conform to your views, then you may find nursing in the community a frustrating experience. On the other hand, for many clients you may become a valued friend and adviser on whose help they rely to maintain a semblance of normal everyday life, and this can be deeply rewarding.

At the time of writing this book, the future organisation of care in the community—and the preparation of nurses (among others) to provide that care—is undergoing radical reconsideration.

The general policy of a speedy return home of those in hospital, the move to community care of the mentally handicapped and the mentally ill, the Cumberlege report advocating neighbourhood nursing schemes, and the Project 2000 recommendations for specialist practitioners—all these and more have highlighted the importance of relevant education and training for nurses in the community, without as yet providing too many answers.

There is a view, for example, that some aspects of the various education programmes for different community specialties might with benefit be merged—so that, say, district nurse and health visitor students all learn some subjects together—and a pilot project has been launched to examine the feasibility of this.

Whatever the outcome of the many initiatives now in hand, it is certain that change in the training of nurses in various community specialties will take years to achieve; so what follows is current practice. If you are using this book to plan your future very far ahead, you should be prepared to expect some changes to have happened in the interim.

District nursing

District nurses provide nursing care for sick people at home, and sometimes in health centres and GPs' surgeries. Their patients include the elderly, the chronically ill, those recently discharged from hospital, the very young and the dying—indeed all those who need the skills of a nurse. They also provide support and advice to those caring for the sick at home, and the health education of the sick and their carers is an important part of the district nurse's work. The district nurse visits each patient as often as may be necessary—and this may be just once or every day—to change dressings, to give injections and generally to provide the care needed.

While nursing skills are obviously important, you will need specific personal attributes too, if you are to achieve real success as a district nurse. You will need, for example, the ability to work closely with colleagues in different disciplines within and outside the primary health care team, and to know when to call on them for support. You will need to be able to work within a district nursing team too, sharing concerns, organising your own case load and perhaps supervising that of others.

You must never forget that you are in the patient's home as a guest, probably a welcome one but even the most welcome guest must not take control unless specifically invited to do so.

There will be many occasions when the temptation to change a patient's lifestyle will be overwhelming. You must be able to distinguish what could be changed from what must be changed—and then have the tact and patience to implement such change to the patient's satisfaction.

Many of your patients will necessarily be elderly, often living alone, sometimes in squalor. For some, your visit will be an expected highlight of the day; others may find it a nuisance, or perhaps not understand at all who you are or why you have come, but all must receive the best of your attention and care. You must learn to listen and to recognise unvoiced pleas for help and counsel.

You will need an even and cheerful temperament, patience, tact and flexibility of attitude. Incidentally, you also need to be able to drive—and you may very well have to provide your own car, claiming reimbursement of costs incurred at a set mileage rate.

Qualification

To be accepted for district nursing training, you must have your SRN or RGN qualification, and some training schools prefer you to have had some experience as a qualified nurse in hospital before they will accept you for the district nursing certificate course.

The course lasts for 9 months, part of which is spent in an establishment of higher education, learning such subjects as psychology and epidemiology, counselling and teaching skills, and consolidating your abilities to plan, carry out and evaluate care, and part of which is spent in supervised practice on the district under the supervision of a practical work teacher—a district nurse who has herself undergone further training in teaching skills. Unlike student nurses, district nurse students are supernumerary.

The final examination includes a written paper on the principles and practice of district nursing, together with assessments of specified work undertaken during the course, assessment of taught practice and assessment of supervised practice.

Once you have passed, you will receive the DNCert.

Funding

The cost of training a district nurse together with her salary while she is training are met by the district health authority where she intends to work after qualifying. If for any reason you find it difficult to persuade your own health authority to fund your training, or you cannot get a training place, it is worth contacting other authorities, provided that you are prepared to move, of course. You should apply in good time—certainly several months before the course is due to start.

The district enrolled nurse

If you are an enrolled nurse, you can also train to work as a member of the district nursing team. In essence, your job will be similar to that of the district nurse once you have qualified, though you will be accountable to her for the care you provide. Training consists of a 16-week course, part of which takes place in an institution of higher education, learning to undertake community nursing duties delegated to you by the district nurse, and part of which is practical training on the district under the supervision of a practical work teacher. The three-part examination includes a written paper on the principles and practice of district nursing, assessment of specified course work and assessment of taught practice. Successful completion leads to the DENCent.

And after that . . .

Once you have consolidated your district nurse training by a period of practice, you may want to do more. If your inclination is to remain with your patients while enlarging or intensifying your own knowledge, you may choose to undertake a course in a relevant specialty, such as stoma care or care of the dying. More and more authorities are now employing district nurse specialists and you should make local enquiries if this appeals to you.

Alternatively, you might apply for further training as a practical work teacher, which will allow you to continue practice while also taking on the practical training and assessment of district nurse students. Later on, you can progress to supervising practical work teaching. If full-time teaching appeals, then you can train as a district nurse tutor. More information about training as an educator appears in Chapter 9 and of course, if your bent is towards organisation, there are management opportunities for district nurses too—see Chapter 10.

Further information

Further information may be obtained from the following:

● National boards for nursing, midwifery and health visiting.
● Queen's Nursing Institute.
● District Nursing Association.
● District Nursing Adviser, Royal College of Nursing.

Health visiting

The skills of those nurses who become health visitors are directed towards promoting good health and preventing illness. This means in essence that the health visitor works as a health educator, both on a one-to-one basis in people's homes and by talking to groups of people in the community. It is her role to foresee potential health problems and to try to intervene to prevent them.

While health visitors work to some extent with every age group, much of the work is with young children and their families, guiding and supporting parents during the early years of childhood.

As much of her work is concerned with anticipating potential problems, a health visitor must always be prepared to learn in order to pass on that knowledge to those who need it, and to initiate support either on her own account or by calling in other professionals in the health, social or education services.

Health visitors do not provide 'hands-on' care. Rather they

are educated to recognise the educational, medical and social needs of their clients, elicited by observation and discussion, and then to respond to those needs in the most effective way.

Health visitors may work within a GP practice or within a catchment area.

According to whether she is based in the country, the town or the inner city, the problems and priorities will differ, but always the health visitor is the one who must recognise and order those priorities, concentrating on clients with particular needs while not neglecting those who are apparently coping well.

In addition to visiting prospective parents, families with new babies and pre-school children and families in their own homes, and carrying out regulation hearing and developmental checks, health visitors may routinely organise baby clinics and mother-and-toddler clubs and set up other support groups as they see the need. It is very much a job of recognising and responding to clients' needs, often unspoken and perhaps unrecognised by the clients themselves, in an attempt to promote family—and community—health.

Health visiting is a challenging job. If you are thinking of training as a health visitor, you must be sure that you are able to get on well with all sorts of people. You will need a great deal of tact, patience and perseverance. You must have initiative and compassion—and you must always be prepared to keep abreast of professional and social developments which may affect your clients' lives.

You will be part of the multi-disciplinary primary health care team and probably leader of a part of it, and maintaining a good open relationship with professional colleagues is important.

You must be able to plan and organise—and you will probably need to be a car driver.

The role of the health visitor is not always very clearly under-stood by the public—and the view that she is simply an inter-fering busybody is still held by a few people in every stratum of society. Nevertheless you will have a duty to visit and to continue to visit even, perhaps especially, those who do all they can to avoid you. If you are the kind of person who shrinks from potentially unpleasant encounters or who takes rejection of your role as rejection of you personally, then health visiting may prove stressful.

On the plus side, there is no doubt that the guidance and support—the reliable friendship—of the health visitor is a rock to cling to for many families caught up in the swirling currents of today's stressful society. If you are strong yourself, there is an enormous satisfaction in sharing that strength with those who need it.

Qualifications

To satisfy the entry requirements for a course in health visiting is currently the first test of the potential health visitor's initiative and determination. You must be an RGN (or SRN). You must also be an RM (or have passed the first part of the old midwifery syllabus) or have completed an approved 12-week obstetric nursing course. These requirements are now under review, and may soon change. Keep your eyes open for news.

If you decide to enter via the midwifery training route, do not announce at interview for midwifery training that you intend to take it in order to become eligible for health visitor training. You will not get in.

If you choose the obstetric course route, you may well have to juggle the times and applications as the course is open only to those already accepted for health visitor training, and for secondment (see later). Health visitor training is a popular option, and you must think about applying for a college place at least a year in advance.

You also need five O levels, or five grade-1 CSEs, one of which must be in English, Welsh or history, or equivalent educational qualifications. Some establishments may require more, and some will expect you to have completed a certain amount of post-registration nursing experience. You will achieve most of this while waiting for your course to start.

Degree courses with a health visiting option are available in three centres, and modified health visiting courses for graduate nurses can also be found. But you will still have to satisfy that midwifery—obstetric training requirement.

The health visiting course lasts a full year and is based in a college of higher education or similar establishment. During your time there, you will study the principles and practice of health visiting, together with social aspects of health and disease, human development, social policy and administration. You will learn aspects of management and research, communication, assessment and teaching skills.

You will also obtain practical experience in the field, under the guidance of a field-work teacher (herself a health visitor who has undergone further training) throughout the academic year. The reports of the field-work teacher to the college will be assessed and at the end of the academic year you will be expected to pass written examinations. You must then embark on a period (9–12 weeks) of supervised practice during which you will have your own case load—and your own mentor. After that you will undergo an oral examination, based on the health visiting studies you will be required to write during the academic year.

If your supervised practice and your examination results are satisfactory, you can then apply to the UKCC to become an RHV—and start to practise.

Funding

Health visitor students are usually seconded to or sponsored on their courses by a health authority. Naturally enough, the health authority will wish to get some return on its investment, and you will normally be expected to work after qualification within the district paying for your training.

So, though you can apply to any health district for secondment (and some do advertise for potential trainees in the nursing press), you must bear your own obligations in mind if you accept an offer.

Secondment includes the fee for the course, together with a salary during training related to your previous position.

You should apply to the director of community nursing services in the appropriate authority and, at about the same time, you should apply to the college for a course place, as the two are interdependent to some extent—and remember you need acceptance by both before you can start your necessary obstetric course. Remember to do it all in very good time, at least 12 months ahead.

It is possible to fund yourself on a health visiting course—perhaps with the help of a local education grant or scholarship if you are lucky enough to get one. Details can be obtained from your local education authority (grants) or from the Community Nursing Association (Royal College of Nursing) or from the Health Visitors Association.

And after that ...

Once you have qualified as a health visitor and begun to practise, you can undertake further short courses in specialist areas either of particular interest to you or of relevance to your work. Refresher courses for health visitors are also available.

Once you have achieved 2 years' experience or more, you can undertake training as a field-work teacher (see Chapter 9), and then yourself become responsible for the practical training of health visitor students, while still practising as a health visitor.

Or you can yourself undertake further full-time training to become a lecturer in health visiting in a college of higher education (see Chapter 9).

Your other way ahead is into management, to become a director of nursing services (community) — or, of course, beyond (see Chapter 10).

Further information

For further information, the following can be contacted:

- National boards for nursing, midwifery and health visiting.
- UKCC Professional Officer (Health Visiting).
- Health Visitors Association.
- Community Nursing Association (Royal College of Nursing).

School nursing

The school nurse has a vital role in enabling children to benefit as far as possible from their education. She is involved in both health surveillance and health education for schoolchildren of all ages.

Sadly a vestige of the old 'nitty Norah' image remains in the minds of some people but this is far from the truth. Today's school nursing service provides help and advice for teachers, families and the children themselves on all aspects of child development.

The school nurse must be aware of the possible effect of health disorders of all kinds on a child's learning capacity and, with the current emphasis on placing children with special needs into the regular education system, she has a special role in advising teachers how their particular difficulties may be overcome.

The school nurse is a member of the primary health care team, but she is an essential part of the school team too.

As part of the primary health care team, possibly under the leadership of a health visitor, she may know in advance of some children with particular problems whom she will see for the first time in the school environment, where new aspects of the old problems may become apparent. Alternatively, she may find that her assessment of children in school will reveal entirely new problems, hitherto unsuspected by parents and other health care professionals.

In any case, she may find herself visiting parents at home to discuss aspects of their children's health care, and this is an important part of her work.

Within the school itself, her involvement will vary according to the views of the head teacher. Some school nurses are deeply involved with teachers in an advisory capacity, offering information on many aspects of health care for the children. They may attend parents' evenings or PTA groups and organise group or individual counselling sessions for the children on such subjects as smoking, obesity and drugs. Unfortunately, other school nurses with as much to offer are confined to testing sight and hearing and to discussing general hygiene.

Apart from the personal attributes of independence and an open and flexible approach which all community health care workers need, the school nurse must have a special affinity with children.

In order to assess their health care needs in relation to their educational environment, it is important that she be able to create the climate of interested caring for the children as individuals which will allow them to express their health problems. Anyone can spot headlice, but it takes a very special approach to persuade a rebellious teenager to seek help for a drug problem. The school nurse also needs an extra helping of tact in her dealings with adults. For the children's benefit, she must be able to offer their teachers advice in such a way that it will be accepted and acted upon, rather than dismissed as interference with another's preserve.

She must be able to discuss—or attempt to discuss—the children's problems with their parents if that seems relevant.

It is perhaps worth saying that, while school nursing can be an absorbing and certainly worthwhile career, it is not an interim in the middle of the main career; rather it is the end of one branch of nursing. If you want to move onwards and upwards, you will have to rejoin general nursing and to undertake further training.

Qualifications

You need an RGN (or SRN) or RSCN qualification to be accepted on a school nursing course.

The courses are organised by health visitor training institutions nationwide and differ widely in presentation—full time, modules, blocks or day release—according to venue, equivalent to about 12 weeks full-time. Part of the course is theoretical, covering child health and paediatrics related to education, and the interaction between the education, health and social service systems, the special needs of the handicapped, child development and the response of children to schooling. The other part of the course is practical and includes some supervised practice. At the end, you will receive a statement of successful completion.

Funding

Aspiring school nurses are seconded by a health authority for training, during which time they receive a salary. If you wish to train, you should apply to the director of nursing services (community) in the district of your choice.

Further information

Further information can be obtained from the following:

- National boards for nursing, midwifery and health visiting.
- Community Nursing Association (Royal College of Nursing).

Practice nursing

Practice nurses—not to be confused with nurse practitioners—are employed by some GPs within their surgeries to undertake nursing duties specified by the GPs themselves.

What this means is that, while some practice nurses have a wide range of nursing duties—immunisation, suturing, health education and organising support groups for patients with problems, for example—and are regarded as valuable members of the general practice team, this is by no means always true.

However, practice nurses themselves are aware of the need to educate GPs in the importance of properly utilising the abilities of the practice nurse and the outlook is improving.

You will need a high degree of competence in the basic nursing tasks, the initiative to identify new areas where your skills could be valuable and the tact to persuade the practice to accept your ideas.

Qualifications

Many GPs require no more than basic nurse training but courses in practice nursing are available in several centres of higher education. Moreover, many of the national board post-basic clinical nursing studies courses (see Chapter 7) are relevant to the work a practice nurse may find herself involved with, depending on the needs of the patients within the practice.

Funding

If you wish to go on a course relevant to your work as a practice nurse, you will have to persuade the practice for which you work to pay for you.

And after that ...

Practice nursing can, in the right environment, be a satisfactory career which you yourself, in partnership with the GPs, enlarge in scope and effectiveness according to perceived needs, but it is not a step forward in a progressive career.

Further information

The following bodies can give you further information:

● National boards for nursing, midwifery and health visiting.
● Practice Nurses' Forum, Community Nursing Association (Royal College of Nursing).

Community psychiatric nursing and community mental handicap nursing

At home with relatives, in small supervised groups in houses or hostels or, sadly, in bed and breakfast accommodation, mentally ill and mentally handicapped people are increasingly being returned to the community.

So there is a corresponding need for nurses with basic training in the care of mentally ill or mentally handicapped people to receive further training to work full time in the community, supporting those discharged from institutional care as they struggle to live in the outside world.

The basic training syllabuses in both these disciplines does include reference to community care, but full-time work in the community requires greater understanding of the family network, of social trends and pressures and of multi-disciplinary teamwork.

The basic characteristics which are needed for any form of community work are needed here, together with tolerance and patience to cope with the hostility you may meet from 'normal' members of the community at large.

Community nurses for the mentally ill and mentally handicapped must be persuasive and determined on behalf of their patients, if those patients are to achieve any sort of satisfactory life in the community setting.

Qualifications

In order to undertake a course in nursing care of the mentally handicapped people in the community or of mentally ill people in the community, it is first necessary to have achieved your basic qualification—RNMH or RMN.

The courses are held in training institutions approved by the national boards and, as these tend to change year by year, you should obtain a current list.

Each course lasts 9 months. That for mental handicap nurses is currently being revised, and the new version will be available from September 1989.

It is recommended that courses are taken before, or as soon as possible after, entering community care.

The courses are intended to prepare nurses to work as skilled practitioners within a multi-disciplinary team, in order to give appropriate care and support to their patients in relation to relevant family and social networks.

Satisfactory completion leads to a certificate in clinical studies.

Funding

You should apply to your manager for secondment to these courses, which will cover both the fees and a salary while you are learning, together perhaps with travelling expenses.

And after that . . .

Further short courses of particular relevance to nurses caring for people with a mental handicap or mental illness are available, as are short refresher courses on current developments.

Or you may wish to undertake further training to enable you to teach full or part time.

As the community services for mentally ill and mentally handicapped people grow and develop, competent caring managers will be increasingly important, and this is a possible area of career development.

Further information

Further information is available from the following:

- National boards for nursing, midwifery and health visiting.
- Mental Handicap Nursing Society (Royal College of Nursing).
- Psychiatric Nursing Society (Royal College of Nursing).
- Community Psychiatric Nurses Association.
- Community Mental Handicap Nurses Association.

CHAPTER 7

Post-basic Clinical Specialties

For many nurses, it would be unthinkable to leave clinical practice, for all the satisfaction and pleasure in their job stem from direct patient care, but clinical practice covers an enormous area, and specialists are needed in many areas of care. Some authorities already employ specialist nurse practitioners, and the proposals of Project 2000 placed emphasis on the need for specialist team leaders.

Undertaking a specialist clinical course need not finally establish your specialist career for ever; many nurses undertake several clinical courses both long and short during a lifetime of nursing. Others stick to their original field and grow ever more capable and knowledgeable.

Some find to their surprise that in the end their clinical expertise does after all lead them away from the bedside into the realms of teaching or research.

Courses to help you to become expert in your chosen field of nursing practice are available, controlled by the national boards, and this is one of the few areas where enrolled nurses are well catered for with some 40 courses designed for them.

Post-basic clinical nursing courses

Under the control of the national boards, syllabuses have been prepared in most fields of clinical nursing practice for courses which are intended to extend and update your knowledge.

You can obtain a full list of such courses from the appropriate

55

national board, but to give you an idea of the variety here is a selection:

- General intensive care.
- Coronary care.
- Renal and urological nursing.
- Neuromedical and neurosurgical nursing.
- Anaesthetic nursing.
- Accident and emergency nursing.
- Orthopaedic nursing.
- Oncological nursing.
- Continuing care of the dying patient and family.
- Rheumatic diseases.
- Psychosexual counselling.
- Alcohol dependency.
- Psychodynamic techniques.
- Behaviour modification in mental handicap.
- Care and management of persons with AIDS.
- Care of the violent individual.
- Child development.

Some of the courses are designed for registered nurses, and some for enrolled nurses; all lead to a nationally recognised qualification.

The courses are of two types.

1. **Certificate courses**: these in general last between 6 months and 1 year and are intended to develop a high degree of professional expertise in the subject covered. Though the courses are designed to prepare you for work in a specialist area, some do require you to have had some (perhaps 6 months') experience post qualification. After successful completion of the course, you will receive a certificate in clinical studies.
2. **Statement courses**: these last between 5 and 30 days (occasionally longer), are intended as updating courses for experienced nurses and concentrate on current practice in the various fields. Successful completion leads to a statement of attendance.

Though controlled by the national boards, these clinical courses are mounted and run by health authorities, often in schools of nursing, and there is a snag. Although the syllabuses for the courses exist, some of the courses themselves in fact do not, because no centre has applied or been approved to put them on. Others are available only in one or two places and, if the course is a popular one, there is strong competition for places, for which local staff may be preferred. In any event, it is wise to apply early. If you are interested in undertaking a specialist clinical course, you should check its current availability with the national boards. The ENB is now computerising its information to provide you with a better service.

Funding

Normally those undertaking these courses are seconded by their own authority; alternatively, you can find out where the courses are held and apply for a job there. In any event, you should discuss your plans with your nurse manager.

Further information

The following should be contacted for further information:

● National boards for nursing, midwifery and health visiting.

Special specialties

It may perhaps seem invidious to pick out three areas of clinical specialisation from so many, but the following have particular points of interest.

Infection control nursing

Like those discussed in the earlier part of this chapter, the foundation course in infection control nursing for RGNs (or SRNs) is controlled by the appropriate national board and leads to the award of a certificate. A certificate is not statutory for practice.

The length of the course is 12 weeks spread over a year, and attendance as soon as possible after entering the field is recommended. Apply to your manager for secondment. Later, you can also attend a shorter refresher course.

What makes this particular specialty so different is the way the infection control nurse works. The role of the infection control nurse is one of prevention and education. She works individually, often based in a microbiology laboratory, with the enormous task of trying to prevent nosocomial infection. The entire hospital environment is hers to monitor—from bedpan washers in the sluice, through disposal of soiled linen, pharaoh's ants in the heat ducts and uncovered cuts in the kitchen—and to improve.

There are not very many infection control nurses—but the few there are have a huge and vital job to do. Their training includes microbiology and epidemiology—and communication, for the essence of their work is the constant encouragement of all staff according to Florence Nightingale's maxim, 'Hospitals should do the sick no harm'.

Further information

● National boards for nursing, midwifery and health visiting.

Occupational health nursing

Hospitals should do their staff no harm either, and it is the occupational health nurse's role to see that they do not.

Curiously, many hospitals have no occupational health service for their staff, and the majority of occupational health nurses are employed outside the NHS. However, occupational health nursing is a legitimate clinical specialty and a few occupational health nurses do find employment within the NHS.

The job includes monitoring the working environment and advising staff and management on possible hazards and how to prevent them, providing emergency care for staff taken ill or injured at work, pre-employment medicals and post-absence rehabilitation. The occupational health nurse may work alone

58

and must be prepared to exercise individual judgement and to take appropriate action, or she may be part of an occupational health team.

At present, there is no statutory requirement for nurses working in occupational health to have any special training at all. One day this may change—and there is a strong body of opinion that it should.

Meanwhile, some outside employers are willing to take on enrolled or registered general nurses without further training, to provide basically a first-aid service.

To do the job properly, as it should be done for the benefit of staff and ultimately management, further training is needed. For the enrolled nurse, an occupational practice course is organised by the English National Board.

For the registered nurse, the training course leads to the award of an OHNC. It lasts 9 months full time or 18 months day release, plus study blocks in an approved centre of higher education. However you do it, the course includes practical experience at the workplace. You need at least 2 years' post-registration experience before you are eligible for the course. You should apply to your employer for secondment if appropriate, and to the centre of your choice for a place (a list of centres may be obtained from the appropriate national board). A diploma course will be available in Aberdeen from September, 1988.

It is perhaps worth mentioning that while occupational health nurses employed by the NHS have the same terms and conditions as other NHS nurses, the majority in the independent sector do not. This may have advantages (possibly higher salary or better conditions) or it may not (less secure and with different pension arrangements).

Further information

Further information is available from the following:

- National boards for nursing, midwifery and health visiting.
- Society of Occupational Health Nursing (Royal College of Nursing).

Ophthalmic nursing

Nursing people with eye injuries or eye diseases not surprisingly calls for particularly meticulous and precise care.

For nurses who have these qualities, a 9-month course is available at ophthalmic nurse training schools countrywide.

The course for enrolled nurses leads to the Ophthalmic Proficiency Certificate, and that for registered nurses to the Ophthalmic Nursing Diploma.

If you wish to be considered for the course, you should apply direct to the school you prefer.

Further information

You should contact the following for further information:

● National boards for nursing, midwifery and health visiting.

CHAPTER 8

Higher Education

In previous chapters, formal education courses which are intended to equip you to practise in a specialised area of nursing have been discussed.

Here we examine diploma and degree courses which will not only extend your knowledge of nursing but also broaden the base of your general understanding and ability to study, to learn, to investigate and to comprehend.

They are designed to stretch your capabilities, and they will do so. You must be prepared for much sustained hard work if you are contemplating entering higher education. The rewards are concomitantly great; you will achieve the satisfaction of personal growth and self-esteem, and a generally more informed approach to your work in future.

On the whole, courses in the higher education sector are concerned with a broader sweep of education than the cramming into your brain of a number of essential facts.

They are more concerned with helping you to comprehend broad concepts, philosophies and theories and with teaching you to begin to formulate your own. They teach you how to gather information, how to sift and analyse it, how to recognise fallacy and irrelevancy and, finally, how to present your own views clearly, supported by the research of others. In other words, they teach you to think for yourself.

This means that, while they include formal lectures, such courses also require you both to participate in discussions with tutors and fellow course members and to read around your subjects at your own initiative in order to expand your ideas by discovering the ideas of others.

The tutors will offer guidelines, but they will not tell you exactly what to do. Essays and projects will be required from you which encompass your own original thought. This can be daunting, particularly to nurses who are too often discouraged from questioning established practice, but it is exhilarating too to be accepted within a peer group as a person whose opinions are worth listening to. You may be contradicted and proved wrong, but at least you will be taken seriously.

However, it is also worth saying that, while patients and colleagues may benefit from your wider understanding, you may well not benefit yourself in terms of recognition. Unless you are or intend to be a teacher, your diploma or degree may be of little or no immediate value. Indeed you will almost certainly meet colleagues who firmly adhere to the view that diploma and degree courses have no place in nursing. However, such ideas are slowly giving place to the more enlightened view that achieving any sort of higher education at the very least reveals qualities of intellectual ability and determination which the profession greatly needs.

If you intend to move ahead in your nursing career, then obviously the higher you go the more important it is to show evidence of such abilities.

However, before you start, make sure you understand your partner's views. You will need support to ensure enough quiet time to study, either at home or at college. Moreover, the entry of one of a pair into higher education can be very threatening to the other who, rightly or wrongly, may feel left behind intellectually and left out of your new acquaintances and activities. Partnerships have foundered on just such difficulties; so do talk it through thoroughly first.

If you are independent, enjoy problem solving and if you are a thinker as well as a doer, then you may well find great satisfaction in the opportunity for exercising your mental abilities which following a course of higher education will give you.

It is said, probably quite correctly, that older people find it difficult to adjust themselves to learning again and that they find it less easy to assimilate and retain new facts than do their younger colleagues, who are more recently attuned to the learning mode. Don't let the fear of failing put you off if your main reason for that fear is age. As very many mature students will tell you, it is perhaps more difficult at first, but you will readjust to the new situation. If you are well motivated, then you will find—and your tutors will help you to find—the study methods that suit you best; mature students have much to offer in terms of determination and sheer experience.

Diploma in nursing

The diploma course is intended to enlarge your understanding of your own nursing field and to equip you to contribute to its development.

The course is organised in six units and takes 3 years of part-time (day-release) study at a college of further education to complete.

In the first year, units 1 and 2 cover the human organism and social organisation and change; in the second year the application of care (unit 3) and the emergence of modern nursing and midwifery (unit 4) are examined; finally, unit 5 examines research and nursing, and unit 6 the search for excellence in your own chosen field. For units 1–4 and 6, your course work will be assessed throughout the year; unit 5 requires you to pass an exam.

On satisfactory completion of the course you will be awarded the Diploma in Nursing from the validating body.

Achievement of the diploma is the most usual route into the Diploma of Nursing Education course which leads in turn to a nurse tutor qualification (see Chapter 9).

To qualify for a place on the course you must have a RGN (or SRN), RSCN, RNMH (or RMNS) or RMN qualification, and you will probably need five O levels (including English Language).

Courses are available at colleges of further education all over the country. Because you will need to take time off (or better still study leave) and to see whether funding is available from your employing authority, you should first approach your nurse manager if you wish to undertake the course. You will also have to find yourself a place by applying to a suitable centre, a list of which can be obtained from the University of London or the appropriate national board.

If you have to fund yourself, you should be thinking in terms of about £300+ per year, which includes registration with the validating body and examination fees. If you have problems with time off, you might consider undertaking the course on your own via the DLC (a correspondence course backed up by local tutorial groups—see Chapter 11).

Advanced Diploma in Midwifery

As the prerequisite to teaching midwifery, or in order to extend your knowledge of the theory and practice of midwifery, you may wish to undertake the Advanced Diploma in Midwifery.

The course examines in depth biology and the behavioural sciences, the theory, psychology and clinical practice of midwifery, the development of the profession and neonatal paediatrics. It lasts 100 days and may be either full time or part time.

Courses are held both in midwifery training schools and in further education establishments throughout the country, and you can obtain a list from the Professional Officer (Midwifery) at the UKCC.

To be eligible, you must have completed 2 years' clinical experience after qualifying as a midwife. Before you apply to the college of your choice, speak to your midwifery manager, who may be able to assist with both the time and the financial help you will need.

Diplomas in management

A number of diplomas in management studies as applied to nursing or the health service in general are available to nurses. For these, some experience in a managerial post is usually required.

These specialist courses are discussed in greater detail in Chapter 10.

First degrees

This book is written primarily for nurses who already have a basic qualification; so I do not propose to cover here those first degrees which lead to registration and a bachelor's degree (plus in some cases a health visiting or district nursing qualification too, after a fourth year of study). Simply, they exist and they are growing in popularity despite the misgivings of the entrenched few.

For the registered nurse in whatever specialty, there are a growing number of degree courses related to nursing available at universities and polytechnics throughout the country, on a full-time or part-time basis.

From October 1987, the Institute of Advanced Nursing Education (Royal College of Nursing), in London, became an affiliated college of the University of Manchester, offering part-time degree courses leading to BSc Nursing Studies or BA Nursing Education.

Full-time course

If you elect to undertake a full-time course, you will of course cease to be employed as a nurse and will thus receive no salary. You can apply for a student grant, however, from your local education authority like any other student. Grants are available for mature students, but it is worth pointing out that, if you are married and your partner is in paid employment, then his or her salary will be taken into account when the amount of your grant (if you get one) is assessed.

Even the full grant is not very much, and from it you will have to pay rent, to eat, to buy books, to pay your travelling expenses and so on. Though nurses' pay is not very high, student grants are even less; so be prepared for a fall in your living standards.

You will of course have the advantage of still being a registered nurse, and so you can think of doing agency work during the vacations. Do ensure that you conform to the conditions of your grant and do not fall foul of the Inland Revenue.

There are currently six centres in the country offering full-time degree courses for registered nurses, one offering a combination, and one a choice. Most of them require other qualifications too. Each of the courses differs in its entry requirements, how to apply, its length and its result. I list the courses here (Table 8.1) but this is simply to give you a flavour of what was available in 1987. Anyone seriously considering pursuing a full-time course should obtain an up-to-date list of courses from the appropriate national board, or consult a suitable reference book.

You must, of course, apply in good time, at least 9 months before the course starts.

Part-time degree courses

Most nurses who undertake degree courses do so on a part-time basis. As with full-time degree courses, what is available changes from year to year; so, if you are contemplating a part-time degree course, then you should find out what is available now. Once again, however, I have given a list of the 1987 courses to give you an idea of the entry requirements, length of course and so on (Table 8.2).

You can choose to study nursing or nursing education or to take a more general course in health studies. For each course, besides your first-level qualification, you will need to show evidence of your ability to undertake the course, usually in the form of a further qualification and/or A levels. Applications for places on part-time courses go direct to the institute concerned.

If you decide that you would like to do a part-time degree course, you should approach your employing authority, who may allow you up to 65 days' paid study leave with expenses.

Just a few lucky nurses each year are accepted for the DHSS degree scheme, which enables you to complete a part-time course, begun on your own initiative, by a year's full-time study usually on full salary plus expenses. For this, you must apply to the DHSS.

Obviously, part-time study is a popular option as it enables you to continue working (provided that your employer allows you the appropriate time off—and these days most authorities do encourage nurses to further their education in this way), but it does take a long time—1 day or evening a week during academic term time for 4 years is the norm.

A few of the part-time degree in nursing studies courses offer

Table 8.1
Full-time courses available in 1987 for registered nurses

Qualifications	Minimum entrance requirements	Further information
Nursing		
BSc (Hons) Nursing Studies 3 years	1. First-level nurse 2. Plus either two A levels or evidence of academic ability Candidates are considered on an individual basis Further nursing qualifications may be taken into account Apply through UCCA	Admissions Tutor Institute of Nursing Studies University of Hull Hull HU6 7RX
BSc (Hons) Nursing Studies 1 year October to September	Candidates should have achieved predominantly A or B grades in all six units of the University of London Extra-mural Diploma in Nursing (revised regulations) In exceptional cases, C grades may be acceptable for one or two first- or second-year units Apply to King's College	Lecturer in Nursing Studies King's College University of London 552 King's Road London SW10 0UA
BSc (Hons) Nursing Studies and the RNT qualification for those who take the education option (full time) 3 years full time or 5 years part time	First-level nurse Education option: must fulfil clinical requirements as laid down by the UKCC for registration as a nurse tutor Candidates with advanced standing may be allowed admission to year 2 of the full-time programme or exemption from parts of the part-time programme, depending on qualifications held Apply to the University of Ulster	Departmental Secretary Department of Nursing and Health Visiting University of Ulster Coleraine County Derry Northern Ireland BT52 1SA

Table 8.1 (*continued*)
Full-time courses available in 1987 for registered nurses

Qualifications	Minimum entrance requirements	Further information
Nursing education		
BA Nursing Education	1. Five GCE passes including two at A level or mature applicants considered on an individual basis	Office of Part-time Education Department of Nursing University of Manchester Stopford Building Oxford Road Manchester M13 9PT
Variable length of course for qualified teachers of nursing, midwifery and health visiting Minimum 3 years or usually 3 years part time followed by 1 year full time for aspiring nurse teachers	2. A qualified teacher of nursing, midwifery or health visiting or aspiring nurse teachers who have satisfied the ENB nurse tutor entry requirements	
	Apply to the University of Manchester	
BA (Hons) Applied Social Science and RHV	1. RGN (or SRN) with midwifery (CBM 1 or SCM (or RM)) or obstetric experience which must be acceptable to the ENB	Course Leader BA (Hons) Applied Social Science Coventry (Lanchester) Polytechnic Priory Street Coventry CV1 5FB
3 years and 1 term	2. In addition, candidates should normally possess one of the following	
	(a) GCE in five subjects, two of which must be at A level	
	(b) GCE in four subjects, three of which must be at A level	
	(c) ONC or OND of sufficient merit	
	(d) Any diploma in higher education of sufficient merit	
	3. Mature students without requirement 2 above may be considered for admission on individual merit	
	Apply through PCAS	

68

BSc (Hons) Occupational Hygiene (Health and Safety at Work)	RGN (or SRN)	Course Director
	BN plus appropriate science-based O or A levels	Centre for Industrial Safety and Health
3 years (4 years if sandwich option followed)	All applications are viewed on individual merit and hence those lacking formal educational–professional qualifications are still encouraged to apply	South Bank Polytechnic Borough Road London SE1 0AA
	Apply to the Polytechnic of the South Bank	
BSc Social Sciences (Health Care Option)	1. GCE O level Maths and *either* two GCE A levels (grades B, C) *or* three GCE A levels (grades C, C, C)	Departmental Secretary Department of Sociology and Social Administration
3 years	2. Candidates aged 21 years or over without requirement 1 above may be considered on individual merit	University of Southampton Southampton SO9 5NH
	Apply through UCCA	
BN	RGN (or SRN)	Director of Nursing Studies
	Candidates' basic education will be considered on an individual basis	University of Wales College of Medicine
3 years		Heath Park
	Apply through UCCA	Cardiff CF4 4XN

Table 8.2
Part-time courses available in 1987 for registered nurses

Qualifications	Minimum entrance requirements	Further information
Nursing		
BSc Nursing Studies 2 years (1 day per week for 33 weeks per year)	First-level nurse plus one of the following 1. Diploma in Professional Studies in Nursing 2. Diploma in Nursing (University of London) 1982 syllabus 3. Diploma in Nursing (University of London) pre-1982 syllabus plus a second qualification requiring at least 1 year of full-time study or equivalent 4. Any other qualification considered by the City of Birmingham Polytechnic to be equivalent to requirement 1, 2 or 3 above	Faculty of Health and Social Sciences City of Birmingham Polytechnic Perry Barr Birmingham B42 2SU
BSc or Diploma in Professional Studies in Nursing BSc takes 4 years Diploma takes 2 years (1 day and evening per week)	1. RGN or SRN 2. A minimum of 2 years' post-registration experience Candidates will normally be required to provide evidence of further academic attainment Holder of the Diploma in Nursing (University of London) may be eligible for exemption of up to 2 years	Course Leader BSc or Diploma in Professional Studies in Nursing Department of Community Studies Brighton Polytechnic Falmer Brighton BN1 9PH

BSc (Hons) Nursing Studies
 	
3 years part time (day release) plus 1 year full time
	1. First-level nurse (UK)
	2. Plus either of the following
	  (a) Two A levels
	  (b) Advanced nursing qualifications, for example RHV, CPN, DNCert, Diploma in Nursing, Diploma in Nursing Education
		Admissions Tutor
		Department of Nursing and Social Studies
		North East Surrey College of Technology
		Reigate Road
		Ewell
		Surrey KT17 3DS

70

Course	Entry requirements	Further information
BSc (Hons) Nursing Studies or Diploma in Professional Studies in Nursing BSc (Hons) takes 4 years but award of Diploma after 2 years (1 day per week for 33 weeks per year)	1. First-level nurse 2. Plus one of the following (a) Two GCE A levels (b) Three SCE H grades (c) Any qualification acceptable to the Leeds Polytechnic	Admissions Officer Leeds Polytechnic Calverley Street Leeds LS1 3HE
BSc Nursing Studies BSc (Hons) Nursing Studies Course consists of modules of approximately 60 hours' teaching per module—equivalent to 2 hours per module per week Modules are taught during day and evening sessions Ten modules at appropriate levels lead to award of BSc with three additional level-4 modules for BSc (Hons) Module credit(s) may be awarded for acceptable qualifications	1. First-level nurse 2. Two A levels or mature entrant selection	Assistant Registrar (Admissions) Institute of Advanced Nursing Education Royal College of Nursing 20 Cavendish Square London W1M 0AB
BSc (Hons) Nursing Studies Variable length depending on number of credits taken each year Minimum 3 years	1. Five GCE passes including two at A level 2. Mature applicants considered on an individual basis	Office of Part-time Education Department of Nursing University of Manchester Stopford Building Oxford Road Manchester M13 9PT

71

Table 8.2 (*continued*)
Part-time courses available in 1987 for registered nurses

Qualifications	Minimum entrance requirements	Further information
BSc (Hons) Nursing Studies 4 years (1 day and evening per week)	First-level nurse Candidates will also be expected to have a recognised post-basic qualification such as Diploma of Nursing (University of London), RHV, OHNC or a certificate granted by the ENB-JBCNS in respect of an advanced course (for example CPN) Nurses without a post-basic qualification will be considered where there is evidence of academic ability Note that a student who successfully completes Part 1 and is unable to proceed to Part 2, becomes eligible for the award of the Diploma in Professional Studies in Nursing on successful completion of a further piece of written work	Course Leader Nursing Section Manchester Polytechnic 799 Wilmslow Road Didsbury Manchester M20 8BR
BSc Nursing Two intermediate levels available: certificate and diploma	2 year's full-time post registration nursing experience May be required to take an entrance test	Course Leader BSc Nursing (Part Time) Department of Molecular and Life Sciences Dundee College of Technology Bell Street Dundee
Nursing education BA Nursing Education BA (Hons) Nursing Education Course consists of modules of	1. First-level nurse 2. A recognised teacher qualification and 3. Two A levels or mature entrant selection	Course Leader Assistant Registrar (Admissions) Institute of Advanced Nursing Education

approximately 60 hours' teaching per module—equivalent to 2 hours per module per week
Modules are taught during day and evening sessions
Ten modules at appropriate levels lead to award of BA with three additional level-4 modules for BA (Hons)
Module credit(s) may be awarded for acceptable qualifications

Multi-disciplinary

BA (Hons) Health Studies (Applied Social Sciences)

4 years part time (1 day and evening per week plus 1 week per year)

1. Three O level and two A level or two O level and three A level passes in the GCE or sit an entrance test and
2. First-level nurse followed by a minimum of 3 years' relevant clinical experience

Course Tutor
Paramedical Sciences
North East London Polytechnic
Romford Road
Stratford
London E15 4LT

BA (Hons) Health Studies

4 years part time (1 full day per week for 30 weeks per year)

1. RGN or SRN
2. Plus an approved qualification of a full- or part-time course of at least 6 months' duration
3. In addition, 2 years' post-qualifying experience in the profession

Academic Registrar
Roehampton Institute
Senate House
Roehampton Lane
London SW15 5PJ

BSc (Hons) Health Studies (Applied Behavioural Science)

4 years part time (day release)

1. First-level nurse
2. 1 years' post-qualifying experience
3. In addition, candidates will normally require one of the following
   (a) GCE in five subjects, two of which must be at A level

Faculty Administrator
Faculty of Community and Social Studies
Newcastle Polytechnic
Newcastle NE1 8ST

Royal College of Nursing
20 Cavendish Square
London W1M 0AB

Table 8.2 (*continued*)
Part-time courses available in 1987 for registered nurses

Qualifications	Minimum entrance requirements	Further information
	(b) GCE in four subjects, three of which must be at A level (c) Any qualification acceptable to the Newcastle Polytechnic, such as a post-registration qualification, for example Diploma of Nursing, RHV 4. Those lacking formal educational qualifications but with an appropriate professional qualification are encouraged to apply as assessment will be on individual merit	
BSc Health Science Studies 4 years part time (1 day per week for 34 weeks per year)	1. First-level nurse 2. Plus 2 years' post-qualifying experience in the profession Minimum age of 23 years	Course Tutor BSc Health Science Studies Department of Life Sciences Nene College Moulton Park Northampton NN2 7AL
BA (Hons) Social Dimensions of Health 4 years part time (2 evenings per week plus 4 days per year)	1. Appropriate nursing qualification 2. Plus a minimum of 2 years' full-time experience in the profession	Course Leader Department of Health Studies Faculty of Education, Health and Welfare Sheffield City Polytechnic 36 Collegiate Crescent Sheffield S1U 2BP

a 'reward' half-way through; for example, the Diploma in Professional Studies in Nursing is both an achievement in itself and acceptable evidence of ability if you wish to take a break half-way and plan to take up your degree again later.

While you are thinking about part-time study, don't forget the Open University. Here you can compile your own programme of courses from an enormous list of subjects and can, of course, choose your own time to study, within limits. More details about the Open University are in Chapter 11.

Higher degrees

If you have acquired, along with your first degree, an overwhelming enthusiasm for higher education — and many nurses do — you can continue your studies, full or part time, by reading for a master's degree (MA, MSc or MPhil) or doctorate (PhD).

Such degrees can be obtained either by a course of learning at an appropriate level, or by choosing, carrying out and writing up a research project on an appropriate topic to an appropriate standard.

Normally, a master's degree will take you 1 year of full-time study or 2 or 3 years of part-time study; a PhD will take longer — 2 or 3 years full time or an equivalent period part time.

There are a number of appropriate courses available in universities throughout the country, and graduate nurses should consult the *Schedule of Postgraduate Courses in UK Universities*, available from the Association of Commonwealth Universities. Most require your first degree to have been a good honours degree.

Once again, employing authorities may offer support, in terms of paid study leave or other funding. You can also apply to your local education authority for funding. If you are undertaking a research-based degree, you may be able to apply for a grant to one of the research councils. Details of grants available are obtainable from the Department of Education and Science.

If you elect to do research to obtain your higher degree — or if your taught degree is in research methods — then you can apply for a DHSS Research Studentship, once you have been accepted as a postgraduate student.

Nursing research

Because much of the research in nursing which is carried on is in pursuit of a degree, this section has been included in this chapter on higher education.

Of course, you do not need to be reading for a degree to elect to be part of the research process.

If you are reading for a higher degree, then you will be allotted a supervisor who will oversee your work to a greater or lesser extent, approving the subject for your research and guiding you through your project to the final preparation of a dissertation.

If you have obtained your second degree, then you may choose to continue in research, attached to a department of nursing within a university, or employed on an individual basis to carry out a specific project of particular relevance to a health authority or within the independent sector.

However, if you are not within the higher education system, don't dismiss the idea of research out of hand.

For many nurses, the very word 'research' calls forth an image of toiling away in dusty obscurity to come up with theories about nursing philosophy which have no apparent relevance to the real world of nursing.

Furthermore, their theses are presented in polysyllables further obscured by incomprehensible jargon.

Nothing could be further from the truth. The findings of nurse researchers often have direct application to patient care and its delivery—or to the conditions of nurses themselves. Nurse researchers on the whole are friendly, talkative people— they have to be if they want to discover views, opinions and facts from other nurses. They have open and enquiring minds and a concern that the practice of nursing is based on fact rather than on myth. For, if nursing is to be taken seriously as a profession in its own right, then research into methods of nursing practice is essential.

Indeed it is the policy of the DHSS to encourage the development of nursing research, and various courses on research appreciation and research methods are offered to those who are interested.

If you are the kind of person who wonders why things happen or are done in the way they are — and is discontented if no reasoned answer is apparent — then you are on the way to appreciating the important role nursing research plays in the profession.

Even if you do not undertake research yourself, awareness of the work of others may help to improve your own patient care. Much research takes place into ways of caring for patients and, if you know about it, then you may be able to put it into practice in your own workplace, citing the research results as the rationale for introducing new methods of care.

What then should you do? First of all, you need to read — the nursing weeklies carry occasional research articles themselves, and more often short accounts of research that has been published elsewhere. Weightier journals carry research papers in full.

Next you might consider enrolling for a course on research appreciation; such short courses are organised by the national boards, the Royal College of Nursing and sometimes by departments of nursing in colleges and universities. The only entry qualification apart from your basic nursing registration is enthusiasm.

Such courses will enlighten you about the need for research, as well as explaining how the network of knowledge thus gained is growing and can be tapped at need.

If you are then inspired to consider undertaking a piece of research yourself, however small, you will need to understand in greater depth the techniques which have to be used in order for your findings to be acceptable. Full- or part-time courses on research methods are held in institutes of higher education but, to undertake such a course, you will probably need to be able to show evidence of higher education yourself: the Diploma in Nursing for example.

Nonetheless, it is worth making contact with a department of nursing if you have a research project in mind, whether or not a course is available to you. You will find advice and support there and perhaps greater help.

There are very occasional openings for nurses to join

established research teams as assistants; there you learn on the job through practical experience.

If you cannot find a course to suit you, think about undertaking one or more of the units which make up the DLC's course on research (see Chapter 11).

A certain number of scholarships and bursaries are available for nurses who wish to gain research experience in a small way. Details are available in the *Directory of Nursing Scholarships, Bursaries and Grants* published by the Royal College of Nursing (which is now rather old) or from the Research Society (Royal College of Nursing).

If you do undertake some research, on however small a scale, do then try to publish your results for the benefit of other nurses in your field nationwide.

You can write up your results for one of the nursing journals, for example. If you choose this route, do study the journals and write your article in the appropriate style. The weeklies adopt a more populist approach to even the most erudite of subjects than does, for example, the *Journal of Advanced Nursing*. It is up to you to select the right one for your own work, which the journal staff will help you to shape once they have accepted your original write-up.

Another method of publicising your results is to present them at a conference. More and more often nowadays, nursing conferences include half-day sessions when the audience splits up into small interest groups who select among a wide choice of sessions presented concurrently. If you see a 'call for papers' within the publicity for any conference, then that is your opportunity to offer your relevant research. Conference organis-ers are on the look out for new talent and refreshing approaches; every abstract is considered simply on the merits of the work it describes and the most obscure have as good a chance as the most famous.

Above all, don't dismiss research as 'not for me'. The results of research projects sooner or later affect the working lives of all nurses whether in practice, in organisation methods or in conditions of service. If you understand more about how the research is carried out, you will gain more yourself from its application.

CHAPTER 9

Teaching

'The students of today are the nurses of tomorrow—and the profession's future is in their hands.' This paraphrase of a well-used public statement is of course literally true.

More realistically, the ability and readiness of today's pre- or post-registration students to contribute to their profession is directly influenced by those who are responsible for preparing them—their teachers.

Teaching is a job which carries great responsibility. Indeed its importance for the future can hardly be overestimated—as the compilers of the report on Project 2000 (see Chapter 3) recognised in their proposals for improving the educational status of teachers. Teaching is hard work but, the report said, it can be greatly fulfilling.

Besides passing on knowledge and skills which is the admitted role of the teacher, it is important to recognise from the beginning that teachers also transmit attitudes to their students. They act, for better or worse, as role models for people who, as insecure learners, are particularly vulnerable to outside influence. The best teachers are enthusiastic, flexible and open minded. They are themselves learning with and from their students. They must always be alert for new ideas and ready to pass them on. Too often, still, we hear of students' disillusion with nursing, and one of the most common complaints is that blind obedience is expected and that a questioning attitude is discouraged. The preparation of nurses to be efficient but unthinking robots is slowly changing—and will have to change if nursing is to have a future as an autonomous profession—but the speed of change is to a great extent in the hands of teachers.

All qualified nurses find themselves taking on a teaching role to some extent, in hospital and in the community, often without specific preparation. All I have said above applies — whether the 'students' are nurse learners or patients or their relatives.

What follows is more specifically directed at those who want to teach an aspect of nursing full time, part time or as a recognised specialist in the field.

With your open-minded attitude must be coupled a real desire to pass on knowledge and skills and the patience to continue to try different ways of doing so — sometimes in the face of what seems intentional non-comprehension.

You must be sympathetic to the aims and aspirations of others, and sensitive to their ideals, even if you do not yourself agree with them. If you do not believe that other people, even when inexperienced, are entitled to their own views and opinions — and may even have original and valuable observations to offer — then you are unlikely to achieve the rapport that a good teacher needs to reach with her pupils.

Nurse tutor

The nurse tutor in general, mental illness, mental handicap and sick children's nursing must be able to prepare and transmit information on a wide range of the theory and practice of nursing in her specialty.

Within a school of nursing, and under the direction of a director of nurse education or senior tutor, she will select the most appropriate methods of teaching particular parts of the recognised syllabus, put such methods into effective practice and evaluate the results, both for the benefit of her students and to maximise the effectiveness of her own teaching practice.

Qualifications

Nurse tutor courses are held in establishments of higher education — universities, polytechnics and colleges of higher and further education. To be eligible for acceptance on a nurse tutor course, you must have had at least 3 years' full-time appropriate nursing experience within the past 7 years, at least 2 years of

80

which must have been at staff nurse level or above, in an area approved for nurse training by a national board. You must also meet the entry requirements of the college you wish to enter.

Moreover you must have completed an approved post-registration course of study equivalent to 6 months full time in the appropriate specialty. Most often this is, in practice, the Diploma in Nursing (see Chapter 8)—though more frequently nowadays nurses are undertaking part-time degree courses (see Chapter 8) as a preliminary to tutor training, and at least one university—University of Manchester—offers a joint BSc–RNT course, and a BA Nursing Education which includes the RNT certificate.

If you believe you are eligible, you should approach the director of nurse education in your own health district. She should confirm both your eligibility and your suitability for tutor training on a form which you must then attach to your application for a place at the college you have selected.

The nurse tutor course comes in different packages, all of which take place in institutions of higher education: as a 1-year full-time course or a 2-year part-time course, or a four-term sandwich course, though the last is available at only one centre. A list of the centres offering the course is available from the appropriate national board.

If you already hold a teaching qualification from a college not approved by the national boards and have achieved the appropriate nursing experience and post-registration course of study, you can apply to the UKCC to have your teaching qualification recorded after 1 year's supervised teaching of student nurses.

In the full-time course, classroom teaching will include the history, theory and practice of teaching as well as sessions consolidating your knowledge of nursing in general. You will also spend some time gaining practical teaching experience in schools of nursing, where you will be supervised by an experienced tutor. She will advise and support you during the practice period and will report on your progress to the college.

If you plan to take a part-time course, you must be already working in a school of nursing (as an unqualified teacher) where once again an experienced tutor will be allocated as your guide and supervisor. You will attend college on a day-release basis, and it is to the college that your supervisor will report on your development.

Both full-time and part-time courses include a specialist unit of study relevant to nurse education.

On satisfactory completion of the course your qualification as a nurse tutor will be recorded with the UKCC, and you will have achieved a Diploma in Nursing Education or a Certificate of Nursing Education, according to where you studied.

Funding

If you are accepted for tutor training, your salary, course fees and certain expenses will be paid by the appropriate national board, which approves a certain number of places in each training institution each year. Once you have been accepted for training by an approved college, then the funding is automatic.

Do apply in good time for all the arrangements to be made satisfactorily before the academic year begins.

And after that ...

After you have qualified as a tutor and gained some years' experience in a school of nursing, you might feel ready to apply for a senior tutor post, eventually progressing to assistant director of nurse education, and finally director.

You may find you also want to specialise in a particular subject or group of subjects. Besides teaching students to registration level, many schools of nursing have undertaken the need to provide continuing education of various sorts for nurses in post. They offer professional development courses and seminars with internal and outside speakers, on clinical and managerial topics; they also provide study days on specific topics such as assertiveness, counselling and so forth, and this trend is increasing nationwide. Nurse tutors who are able and willing to organise such courses are always in demand.

Some schools are approved centres for various national board courses on nursing specialties (see Chapter 7) and you may choose to become involved with setting up one of these.

Project 2000 (see Chapter 3) has highlighted the desire of many nurse tutors themselves to seek higher qualifications. If you did not enter teaching via the degree route, you may now be offered the opportunity to achieve one part-time—or to read for a master's degree if that is appropriate.

Innovatory work in course design and curriculum development is possible.

Further information

Further information may be obtained from the following:

- National boards for nursing, midwifery and health visiting.
- Institute of Advanced Nursing Education (Royal College of Nursing).
- Your own director of nurse education.

Clinical nurse teacher

An RCNT was responsible for teaching students the practical nursing skills in general, mental handicap, mental illness or sick children's nursing. She did so by explanation, demonstration and supervision of practice both in the classroom and, when the students were not in school, in the wards.

However, late in 1987, training of clinical teachers ceased and will not be resumed. All nurse training is now undertaken by nurse tutors, sometimes with unqualified helpers who themselves wait for tutor training.

Midwife teachers

As a midwife teacher you will be responsible for preparing student midwives in the art and science of midwifery, so that they may acquire the skills and confidence to practise independently. You will be based in a school of midwifery and will be responsible for the students' overall progress. This will include liaison with the community midwives under whose supervision the students obtain their community experience.

Qualifications

If you want to become a midwife teacher, you need first to obtain the Advanced Diploma in Midwifery (see Chapter 8), and you must work as a midwife for the 12 months immediately preceding the teaching course. If you think you are eligible, approach first your local midwifery manager, before applying to a college.

It is a 1-year full-time course, held at a university or college of further education. A list of colleges can be obtained from the appropriate national board.

On the course, you will consolidate your knowledge and practice of midwifery under the supervision of a midwifery teacher, but other parts of the course which cover education theory and practice and subjects such as sociology, epidemiology, counselling, care planning and so on are likely to be shared by students in other disciplines, such as aspiring health visitor and district nurse tutors.

You will also gain practical teaching experience at a school of midwifery supervised by an experienced midwife teacher.

Funding

Local health authority funding may or may not be available; so your first approach should be to your midwifery manager.

And after that . . .

Once you have qualified as a midwife teacher and have gained experience, you can choose to progress upwards to senior tutor. You can elect to specialise and extend your knowledge of a particular branch of midwifery, organising refresher and professional development courses for qualified midwives in your district. You can continue your own education to degree level and beyond. You might even do all these things simultaneously.

Further information

The following will supply further information:

- National boards for nursing, midwifery and health visiting.
- Your local midwifery manager.
- Royal College of Midwives.
- Midwifery Adviser, Royal College of Nursing.

District nurse tutors and lecturers in health visiting

Full-time (and sometimes part-time) teachers of health visiting and district nursing are based in institutes of further education and are responsible for organising and providing their students with the formal education making up the health visitor and district nurse courses.

They often work together, within a 'department of community studies' perhaps, and share responsibility for those aspects of the curriculum the two specialties have in common—sociological studies, family dynamics, organisation of the health services and so on. Others are responsible for teaching the individual aspects of the specialties.

Tutors and lecturers are also responsible for liaison with those practitioners who are designated teachers in the community and who supervise the practical part of the students' learning experience, and for coordinating all aspects of the course.

Qualifications

If you are interested in becoming a teacher in district nursing or health visiting, you will need to have at least 2 years' experience as a qualified district nurse or health visitor.

The course is full time for a year and is held in a university or institute of further education. A list of approved centres is available from the national boards.

Besides consolidating your own professional skills, the course will cover theory and practice of education and teaching, coordination of a training programme, administration and organisation within further education and, of course, teaching practice under supervision.

Part of your learning will take place in mixed-specialty groups, some only with colleagues from your own specialty.

Once you have completed the course successfully, you will be awarded the District Nurse Tutor Certificate or Health Visitor Tutor Certificate.

Funding

Before you apply for a place at your chosen college, discuss the availability of funding with your community nursing manager.

And after that ...

The way is now open for you to progress to senior tutor (or lecturer) and eventually to head of department.

Further information

Further information is available from the following:

- National boards for nursing, midwifery and health visiting.
- Your own community nursing manager.
- Health Visitors Association.
- Community Nursing Association (Royal College of Nursing).

Practical work teachers (district nursing) and field-work teachers (health visiting)

If you are interested in pursuing a teaching role but at the same time want to continue as a practising district nurse or health visitor, then you might like to consider training as a district nursing practical work teacher or health visiting field-work teacher.

As such, you will be allocated a number of students who will come to you for their community experience. You will be responsible for providing them with as wide a range of experience as possible, teaching and explaining the techniques you use in different circumstances, overseeing their own supervised practice within the community and reporting back on their performance to the college-based tutors. You will continue to practise yourself as a district nurse or health visitor.

District nurses and health visitors who undertake this extra role find it immensely satisfying to be able to continue in direct patient care while at the same time contributing to the future good practice of their profession.

Qualifications

You need to have at least 2 years' experience after qualification as a district nurse or health visitor before applying for the teachers' course.

The course consists of 6 weeks' study at an approved training institution (lists from the appropriate national board), followed by supervised teaching practice. At the end you will receive a Practical Work Teacher Certificate or Field-work Teacher Certificate, as appropriate.

Funding

The health authority who employs you will second you for this training, so long as money is available and teachers needed; so talk to your community nursing manager.

And after that . . .

The next step is to become a supervisor of practical work or field-work teachers—another course leading to greater responsibility for the quality of community experience provided for district nurse or health visitor students.

Further information

Further information can be obtained from the following sources:

- National boards for nursing, midwifery and health visiting.
- Your local community nursing manager.

CHAPTER 10

Management

Contrary to popular myth, managers are not in post to thwart the best intentions of hard-working nurses simply trying to do their job, but it is understandable that people do feel resentful of their managers, for to do the job well requires ability and competency in areas in which many nurse managers have received little or no formal training.

Slowly the situation is changing as responsible health authorities recognise that neither newly qualified nor more experienced nurses feel adequately equipped to undertake the management aspects of their work.

In response to nurses' pleas, professional development courses are starting up which examine areas within the 'management' role, rather than purely clinical aspects of care.

All nurses have some 'management' responsibilities but, once you have qualified, and beyond, the proportion of your working day spent on management tasks increases. If you continue to seek promotion, the day will come when your job is purely a management one, with perhaps a clinical task or two inserted by you simply 'to keep your hand in' so to speak.

If you do aspire to such a post—and indeed to continue perhaps to general management rather than purely nursing management—then there are certain skills which you will need to acquire.

Certainly not all managers have all these skills (and you may never be asked about them at interview), but to become a 'good' manager—to achieve the best possible care for patients by able and motivated staff within budgetary constraints, while retaining the respect of your superiors and peers within the management team—it is essential that you acquire most of them.

Everyone can recognise a poor manager. She is virtually unknown to most of her staff because she rarely leaves her office and speaks only to her peers and superiors. She excuses all shortcomings with 'I wasn't told', and she is a mistress of inaction and procrastination.

To recognise a 'good' manager is harder, but here are some of her essential qualities.

1. A good manager must start by being able to manage herself. If you cannot do that, you cannot hope to be successful in managing others. You must be able to order your day, to set your own priorities and to be flexible enough to change them at need. You must be professionally aware, not only on your own account, but also to enable you to anticipate the needs of your staff. You must be, and be seen to be, competent to cope calmly and effectively with all sorts of people and problems. You must be decisive and take responsibility for your decisions. You must recognise and work on your own weaknesses. If you can at least make a start on all these things, you will be in a position to foster similar abilities in your staff.

2. Skills in communication are essential. You must be able to talk to your own staff, patients and people in other disciplines, in both a formal and an informal way as appropriate. You must also learn to listen. You will be representing nursing at meetings and discussions, and you must learn how to present your case relevantly and clearly. You must learn the art of writing reports so that they will be read—and perhaps even acted upon.

3. To manage people effectively, you must also like them, care about them and respect them. This is not always easy, but a manager who is contemptuous of her staff's abilities or indifferent to their concerns can never create the right climate for them to learn and develop. You must recognise when praise is more effective than reprimand (and vice versa). You must not shrink from conveying unpleasant but essential truths but you must learn the best way, time and place to tell them. You must also recognise, accept and act upon unpleasant truths which are told to you. An effective manager will forge links between herself and her staff and

between herself and her own manager, enabling a constant two-way exchange of information both major and minor to occur. She will know what to tell, who to tell and when to tell, and so will the others. Only if you know what is going on in all aspects of your working life can you be in any position to control the outcome.

4. As their manager, you are responsible for the standards achieved by your staff and you must do all you can to maintain and improve them. Once again, this means creating a climate for learning and motivating staff to take every opportunity to improve. It does not mean setting impossible goals; you must encourage staff to set and achieve reasonable objectives and then move on to greater efforts.

5. All these factors are set in a climate of financial restraint. Whatever you may think of the health service financing, you cannot ignore the fact that the amount of cash available is limited. While you may not yourself be accountable for an allocated budget, all the same you are, in the interests of your patients, responsible for not wasting it. So it is sensible to understand a little about what there is and where it goes. There is no virtue in ignoring or dismissing finance as of no relevance to caring. It is relevant, if only that its lack prevents you doing what you want. If you can learn how the money side of your job works, you are in a better position to manipulate it to achieve the best possible patient care.

Don't let all these imperatives put you off if you feel inclined towards a career in management. Most nurses have the ability to encompass and practise all these skills—indeed you may already be using some of them in your day-to-day work. However, to become a good manager you need some extra help to recognise the skills you have and to use them effectively—and to start to accumulate those you do not have.

As I said earlier in the chapter, you may never be asked at interview whether you possess all or any of these skills, and it is certain that many managers do not. Nevertheless, once you are in post, your abilities in these areas will become apparent and, if you are hoping for further promotion in future, then you will need to show evidence of capability in terms of successful managing in the job you already have.

The spotlight in the health service has fallen squarely on management with the implementation of the Griffiths recommendations, and the failure of nurses to secure general management posts in the first round of appointments has helped to highlight shortcomings in the education and training of nurses in that important area.

To ensure a strong voice for nursing in the health service of the future, it is essential that aspiring nurse managers—as well as those already in post—grasp every opportunity to improve their management skills in order to hold their own in the tough competition for top jobs.

So what can you do to improve your own chance of securing a management post and performing well in it?

First of all, grasp any opportunity that may be offered by your health authority to improve any aspects of the skills I have listed earlier.

Forward-looking authorities do now offer study days or short courses in various techniques allied to management but, if yours is not one of these, it would do no harm to ask whether a course on, say, communication skills or assertiveness might be organised. You might be surprised to find an enthusiastic response to your request from a tutor or nurse manager who may have already herself tried to get agreement for such a course, to be met by the stonewalling reply that there has been 'no demand' for it.

The skills and techniques of management are basically the same, in whichever context they are used. You may find that your local adult education institute has relevant day or evening courses from which you may learn the skills—which you then have to relate to the health service environment.

You can borrow books from the library on management skills, both related to nursing and set in a wider context—and of course you will maintain your professional awareness by reading the nursing journals, skimming other journals in related disciplines, taking a quality newspaper and attending relevant conferences and seminars whenever you can manage it.

If you undertake a course of advanced nursing education, health visitor training, for example, or the diploma in nursing, you will find it contains elements of management techniques.

However, perhaps all this will not be enough for the nurse manager of the future.

Some health authorities do offer first-line management courses, often organised in collaboration with a local college, to nursing staff at sister or charge nurse or district nurse or health visitor level. If yours is one of them, put your name forward for the course as soon as you can.

Middle management courses may be available—often organised by a health district for new managers in different disciplines—and you should apply for those too whenever you are eligible.

You might too, at this sort of level, consider applying for a place on one of the part-time management courses offered by higher education institutes. Such courses differ from place to place in their demands on your time and the entry qualifications; so you will need to find out for yourself what is available locally.

As an aspiring manager, you will need the qualities of self-motivation, fact finding and organisation. Make it your first task to discover a suitable course and to persuade your manager to send you on it.

While you are casting around for courses, try the Institute of Health Service Administrators, the Institute of Personnel Management, the National Staff Committee for Nurses and Midwives and, of course, the Institute of Advanced Nursing Education (Royal College of Nursing).

As an example of the kind of course you might be looking for, the Institute of Advanced Nursing Education offers a 1-year part-time programme in management studies, orientated towards the health service, which is suitable for nurses from ward sister level up. Its successful completion leads to a Royal College of Nursing Certificate in Management Studies, and this is itself part of the entry qualification to the next step—a 1-year course for a Diploma in Management Studies.

Other courses available for more senior staff include the Diploma in Health Services Management, the Diploma in Advanced Nursing Administration (both offered by the Institute of Advanced Nursing Education), master's degree programmes in business studies which are available for nurses with a first degree or other suitable qualifications, and multi-disciplinary courses for senior managers mounted by the NHS Training Authority.

The rewards of a management post are hard to assess. You will be better paid, of course, though probably not so well as your contemporaries in the private sector. For that extra money you will work long hours and bear heavy responsibilities.

You will receive little praise and probably much blame. Nevertheless, you will achieve the satisfaction—if you have done the job properly—of knowing that you have created an environment in which your staff can give of their best and, if they do well, then some of the reflected glory is yours, for recognising abilities and enabling them to flourish.

You will represent nursing—in meetings of the management team and later, perhaps, in public—and, if you perform well, then you will do your profession inestimable service.

Don't neglect to discuss your career development with your own manager while you are considering whether to undertake a course and which to opt for. Your career prospects and ambitions should in any event form part of an ongoing, if irregular, dialogue between you and your manager. If they do not, then you should take the initiative. She should have both up-to-date information and her own experience to guide you— together with knowledge of the kind of help you can expect from your health authority—study leave and/or contribution towards the fee.

For other information, you should contact the organisations whose addresses are given at the end of this book.

CHAPTER 11

Distance Learning

The earlier chapters in this book have described various courses of formal learning available to nurses who want to further their careers in specific directions. However, in this chapter, I shall concentrate on those areas in which an individual can decide for herself to continue her own education under her own steam.

'Distance learning' is simply a new term for the kind of course which you work through at home, in your own time, and to a certain extent at your own speed—a much improved and modernised version of the old 'correspondence course'.

Nowadays, distance learning materials are carefully designed to be easily read and assimilated and make use not only of printed materials but also of cassettes, video tapes and charts— visual aids to learning of every sort.

Self-testing devices are widely used, and some programmes are backed up by a tutorial system which enables you to discuss your problems with a sympathetic 'tutor' and with your peer learners.

There are many good reasons why you might decide to investigate the possibilities of embarking on a course of open learning.

The first is simply to enlarge your own horizons. Courses are available on many health-care topics which, while not directly related to nursing, will nevertheless contribute overall to your ability to practise simply because they introduce you to new ideas and new ways of approaching them.

Other open learning programmes are designed with nurses in mind, and these are intended specifically to update and deepen your knowledge on a particular nursing topic. If you take a longer-term view, it is possible to read for a degree through the

Open University and thus open new horizons for yourself on a wider scale.

One of the proposals of Project 2000 (see Chapter 2) was that continuing education should be available for nurses on a wide scale but that time is not here yet. Indeed the availability of professional development courses of any sort—from single study days organised locally to short courses administered nationally by statutory bodies—leaves a great deal to be desired.

So, if nursing is to develop as a profession, its individual members have to take some responsibility for their own continuing education in the interests of improved patient care and their own job satisfaction and career development. In this context, it may be worthwhile to consider here periodic registration, and what it may entail in future.

Periodic registration

The introduction by the UKCC in January 1987 of a periodic registration fee caused an uproar.

Nurses were outraged at being asked to re-register and at having to pay to do so every 3 years, but this is just the first step in a policy of reform by the UKCC which has as its goal the professional status of nursing by self-regulation.

The long-term intention—and one which will eventually require an amendment to the 1979 Act which establishes the UKCC and national boards—is that, while qualifications will be registered on a lifetime basis, each nurse will be issued with a 'licence to practise' which will be renewed periodically only provided that certain conditions are met.

These conditions will be concerned with proof of professional competence—which is where professional self-regulation comes in. As things stand at present, a nurse once registered can continue as a nurse forever, provided that she does not get struck off for misconduct. There is no further test of competence. Any nurse, however old, out of date, ignorant of new techniques or just plain incompetent, can continue to practise provided that someone will employ her. It is this state of affairs that the UKCC seeks to improve eventually through the introduction of a system which will require practitioners to show evidence to the UKCC of their continuing ability to nurse in today's conditions.

Thus the UKCC will become the body which not only determines entry requirements to the profession but also is wholly and solely responsible for maintaining professional standards at an acceptable level among all practising nurses.

Thus, some time in the future, you too will very probably have to prove that you have maintained your professional competence and knowledge. How, when and where 'mandatory refreshment' (midwives have it already, by the way) will take place is still under discussion (UKCC discussion paper in September 1987). One acceptable way may very well be by showing evidence of having undertaken certain approved distance learning courses.

Commitment

Before you embark on a course of open learning, it is sensible to examine your own workaday life to ensure that you will have both the time and the support to do it.

It may suit you to set aside in advance special times which you will devote to your learning; otherwise, unless you are very strong minded, other (apparently more immediately pressing) concerns will intervene. It is all too easy to put off studying, particularly when you set your own deadlines, so to speak, and have no tutor or peer group to support you – or shame you into doing your work on time.

Of course, if you do drop out half-way through, it will be only your own time and perhaps your own money that you have wasted. Nevertheless, you may also experience a niggling feeling of failure which will do little for your self-esteem. On the other hand, successful completion of an open learning course brings in its wake deserved elation.

Moreover, while prospective employers will not know about your failures, they will be impressed by your achievements if you are able to show that you have successfully completed such a course. It is a view increasingly held that to have undertaken an open-learning course reveals candidates not only to be slightly more knowledgeable in whatever field, but also to have

97

other useful attributes—persistence, self-responsibility and ambition—all of which accumulate for you extra points in the battle for promotion or for a place on a popular course. Some distance learning material is specifically designed to be undertaken by a group, who will provide support for each other and opportunities for discussion under the leadership of a group tutor. Other courses are simply for individuals—and it is for these that you must be particularly well motivated and self-supporting.

If you do intend to undertake a personal course, you might consider enlisting the interest of one of the tutors in your local school of nursing or your nursing manager. It is sometimes useful to be able to discuss issues with a more experienced person rather than those at the same level as you; nurses with teaching or managerial experience may be able to throw new light or offer ideas which may not have occurred to you on a purely informal basis. However, only you can decide whether such a helpful other person exists in your district.

Funding

Most people who embark on a course of open learning are prepared to fund themselves—and courses are priced with that in mind.

Most short courses cost between £20 and £30. However, if even that is too much for you, then it is worth approaching your school of nursing to see whether they would be prepared to fund you as an individual or even consider taking on a group project. Be prepared for a refusal, though you may be surprised to discover a little-known fund available for just such individual projects. It is always worth asking.

An Open University degree

Though greeted with some cynicism when it was first established in 1969, the Open University has proved itself beyond all doubt – and has set standards in the open learning materials it produces which publishers of standard educational texts are still striving to emulate.

The Open University offers BA degree courses which are unique in the UK. You need no formal educational qualifications to take the course; you can to a large extent select your own broad areas of study, and of course you work in your own home at the times which suit you best.

The Open University provides about 130 different courses, at varying levels of difficulty. Each course lasts 9 months (February to October), and each is rated as a 'credit' or 'half-credit'. Credit courses, on the whole, demand about 14 hours of study each week, and half-credits about 14 hours a fortnight. To achieve a BA degree from the Open University, you must accumulate a total of six credits (eight for an honours degree).

If you have successfully completed at least 6 months' full-time study at a higher educational level you may be eligible for the award of credit exemptions, which will cut down the number of Open University credit courses you must complete for your degree. However, basic nurse training (RGN (or SRN), RMN, RNMS and RSCN) will not give you an exemption. If that is all you have, you must complete the full six credits. Each claim for exemption is treated individually; so you should write formally to request exemption if you think you are eligible.

Courses are available at 'foundation' level and then at second, third and fourth levels of difficulty.

Foundation courses exist in the Faculties of Arts, Mathematics, Science, Social Sciences and Technology. The School of Education does not offer a foundation course but, once you have achieved foundation level in another faculty, you can go on to take a course at second level from the education list.

You must start your degree study with a foundation course (one credit) and you must successfully complete a foundation course from another faculty at some time within your accumulation of six credits. The rest of the six credits can be a combination of credit or half-credit courses at second level from any of the faculties. Restrictions on combinations of courses within a degree programme are kept to a minimum; so you are free to construct your own programme of study depending on your individual needs and interests.

You can choose to take anything from a minimum of one half-credit course to two full-credit courses in 1 year—or you can put your degree 'on ice', so to speak, and take a year or more off in the middle.

If you plan an honours degree, then at least two of your eight credits must be at third or fourth level.

The Open University is adding to its list of courses all the time, but credit and half-credit courses at various levels are available on many specialised topics with such broad groupings as the following: art; history; biology; chemistry; classical studies; computing and computers; design; earth sciences; economics; education and society; psychology of education; educational policy; management and curriculum development; electronics; engineering design; engineering mechanics; European studies; geography; government and politics; history; literature; management; materials; pure mathematics; applied mathematics; methodology; music; philosophy; physics; psychological studies; public administration; religious studies; applied social studies; sociology; statistics; systems; twentieth-century studies.

How you select the courses to make up your individual degree programme will depend to a great extent on why you are doing it and where your particular interests and ambitions lie.

Each course consists of 'units' which reach you through the post. They contain material to read, notes on set books, and notes on radio and television broadcasts related to your particular course. For some courses, you may also receive audiovisual material and returnable scientific equipment to do your own experiments. You will be required to submit your own work for assessment. You will be allocated to a tutor who will help and advise you throughout the course, and you can attend a local study centre (there are 250 nationally) to talk both to your tutor and to fellow students following the same course.

All foundation courses and some others require your attendance at a 1-week residential summer school held at a university during the summer vacation.

At the end of the course, you will take a written examination, and your performance in this together with some of the assignments you have completed throughout the course will determine whether you achieve the credit for which you have been working.

The application period for the Open University degree programme closes approximately 6 months before the course starts, in other words in September for the next February, but it is advisable to apply as early as you can because the places are limited. The Open University starts to offer places from April of the preceding year; so applying a year in advance is sensible. You need no formal educational qualifications, but you must be at least 18 years old and resident in the UK when the course starts.

Although the Open University does administer a certain amount of funds to help students who cannot afford to study, or to continue to study, you should be prepared to fund yourself. You can pay by instalments. You should budget for about £200 for a foundation course, £100 for a half-credit course and £125 for summer school.

Further information is available from the Open University whose address you will find at the end of this book.

Diploma in Nursing

The Diploma in Nursing (see Chapter 8), which is a prerequisite for some further formal education courses (see, for example, Chapter 9) has until recently been available only as a course requiring part-time attendance at an approved institute of higher education.

This has meant that some aspiring students unable to obtain day release, or to travel to an appropriate centre, have been prevented from taking the course.

Now, however, a distance learning package is available, backed by tuition, counselling and library facilities in designated local study centres throughout the country. The learning materials are prepared and despatched by the DLC (which comes under the auspices of the Department of Nursing and Community Health Studies, at the South Bank Polytechnic) and the course is validated by the University of London.

The course takes 3 years to complete, each year based on 38 study weeks and requiring a minimum of 180 hours of formal study, together with extra reading time and at least six half-day sessions at the local study centre. In other words, you will need to set aside perhaps 10 hours a week for studying, as well as six mornings, afternoons or evenings during the year.

Each year you will undertake two units of study (90 hours each); in year 1, the units cover the biological, psychological and social sciences as they affect nursing practice; year 2 examines theories and concepts of nursing and how they are applied to care (unit 3), and the development of modern nursing and midwifery and the roles and responsibility of the nurse in society (unit 4). In the final year, you are required to focus on a chosen area of study, to demonstrate an appreciation of research methods (unit 5) and to describe both innovations in practice and evidence of a search for excellence in nursing (unit 6).

In each of the first 2 years, you will be required to submit six pieces of written work for assessment. In the third year, you have to undergo a 3-hour written examination for unit 5 and to submit two papers for unit 6.

During each year of the course you receive regular mailings of study material from the DLC, including a workfile, 'blocks' of printed text, and other learning aids as appropriate.

What you learn from these is of course consolidated by sessions at the local study centre, including face-to-face tuition, and discussions with both tutor and fellow students.

You must be a registered nurse to undertake the course, and normally you will be required to have five O levels, one of which must be English or Welsh Language.

The courses start in September each year and you must apply in good time to your local study centre, who will carry out initial selection procedures. Application forms are available through the local centres but, if you do not know of one, the DLC will send you a list—their address is at the back of the book.

If your employer will not fund you—and you should certainly ask your director of nursing services or director of nursing education first—then you might consider whether to fund yourself. As well as the cost of the course materials (currently (1988) £14.75 per block), you will have to pay the registration and assessment fees of the University of London, postage for your essays, stationery and travel expenses.

Further information is available from the DLC or your local study centre.

Short courses

As the concept of distance learning as a valuable addition to more formal methods of teaching becomes widely accepted, so too has grown the variety and level of distance learning material available, and much more is being produced.

Some of the short courses available have been specifically designed for nurses; others are intended for a wider audience of health care professionals.

They have in common the open learning system that enables you to progress very much at your own pace, and to work in the way that best suits you. You are in control.

That said, it is much easier to study within the supportive framework of an informal group of like-minded people. If you are thinking of undertaking a short course, do enquire of your local school of nursing (ask for the continuing education tutor or post-basic education tutor) whether she knows of any such group.

No book could hope to cover all the options available to you in such a proliferating field but, to give you some idea of the short courses available for nurses, the outputs of two pioneering groups, both established in 1984 under the Open Tech Programme of the Manpower Services Commission, are worth examining.

The DLC at the South Bank Polytechnic is producing a series of study packs under the general heading 'Managing care'.

Each of the study packs is so designed that an individual nurse, working entirely alone and without tutorial help, can achieve the specified learning objectives. Nevertheless, the DLC acknowledges the problems of such isolation; so, to each individual student registered with the DLC, tutorial help is offered through one of its lecturers. Meanwhile, it is also establishing a network of 'open learning coordinators' within schools of nursing, to whom local students can go for information, advice, counselling, coaching, advocacy and feedback.

In some parts of the country, students and/or tutors have

taken the initiative and themselves formed study groups, for support and guidance. If you are interested in any of the DLC courses, enquire from your local school of nursing (continuing or post-basic education tutor) whether such a group exists. Alternatively, the DLC itself may be able to advise you of study groups in your district.

Within the 'Managing care' series, study packs are available on, for example, stress in nursing, teaching patients and clients, being assertive and so forth.

To give you an idea of what you get for your money (in this case £22.50 at the time of going to press), here is a description of 'Being assertive'.

The pack contains a workbook and a reader. The workbook is divided into a number of sections, each of which includes a number of activities through which you can analyse your own knowledge, skills, attitude and approaches and relate the issues and ideas introduced in the study material into your own work area. The sections are as follows:

1. What is assertiveness?
2. Assertive rights and responsibilities.
3. Assertive and non-assertive approaches.
4. Getting your point across . . . and listening.
5. Refusing, negotiating and cooperating.
6. Giving and receiving feedback.
7. Applying assertiveness.

The reader contains a selection of relevant articles and extracts to use in conjunction with the workbook.

Further information about this and the others in the 'Managing care' series is available from the DLC.

The DLC has also produced a programme entitled 'Research awareness', developed to help nurses to understand research in relation to their own practice. It comes in a series of modules, each of which requires about 8–12 hours of study. The DLC anticipates that nurses may buy single, particularly relevant modules for their own use or that tutors may use single modules to illustrate particular areas of teaching. However, some people may undertake the entire thirteen modules and for them tutorial support will be available from the DLC together with a discount on the individual module price of £12.50 (1988).

Under the title 'Continuing nurse education; open learning for nurses', the Colleges of Barnet and Central Manchester have cooperated to produce an interesting series of open learning modules.

Once again each module centres on a well-produced workbook, featuring self-assessment exercises and worked examples. Other helpful information is included as relevant. These courses are intended entirely for your own use; no tutorial help is provided. Once again, you might find it easier if you could discover a partner or group who would undertake the course with you, thus providing support and the chance of discussion. A module costs between £20 and £25. Those currently available include 'Nursing today', 'Measurement in nursing', 'Interpersonal skills', 'The nature of cancer' and 'Management of learning'. More are in preparation.

Here to give you an idea of what the course comprises is the contents list of the 'Nursing today' module.

The workbook consists of the following:

Introduction

Section 1 The nurse as a worker
      1.1 The nursing workforce
      1.2 The social status of nursing
      1.3 A nurse's rights as a worker and a citizen
      1.4 A nurse's rights (other aspects)
      1.5 Labour relations in the National Health Service

Section 2 The nurse as a professional person
      2.1 Professionalism
      2.2 Accountability
      2.3 Legal issues
      2.4 Ethical issues

Section 3 The wider context of health care
      3.1 Health and society
      3.2 Society and nursing
      3.3 The health system
      3.4 Health policy
      3.5 The nursing system

Conclusion

Appendix 1 Florence Nightingale pledge for nurses

Appendix 2 International Council of Nurses Code for Nurses (1973)

Appendix 3 UKCC Code of Professional Conduct (1974)

Appendix 4 American Nurses' Association Revised Code of Ethics

Appendix 5 Editorial, *Nursing Times*, 2 July 1986

Glossary

Acts of Parliament and Official Reports

Bibliography

Index

Further information can be obtained from the Continuing Nurse Education Programme, whose address is at the end of the book.

The Open University's Department of Health and Social Welfare has embarked on a programme of courses directed towards health care professionals in various areas.

Several are already available and there are more being prepared, concentrating on areas of particular current concern and prepared in association with involved professionals.

In general, the courses are prepared for undertaking by groups of people, who work individually with their own study packages, then come together for group discussion and participation under a leader.

Courses currently available are as follows:

- Abuse in families.
- A systematic approach to nursing care.
- Mental handicap: patterns for living.
- Rehabilitation.

- Caring for older people.
- Caring for children and young people.
- Coronary heart disease.

To give you an idea of what the courses are like, what follows is a description of the coronary heart disease course, the first in the series 'Education for health', aimed at all members of the primary health care team and put together in association with the Health Education Council.

'The course aims to help primary health care workers—GPs, practice nurses, health visitors and community nurses—to improve their understanding of the risk factors in coronary heart disease and the potential for reducing these risks, and to promote planned coordinated action.

The course will also be relevant to wider secondary audiences concerned with health promotion.'

The individual study pack (£35) contains the following:

- A workbook—the main study text.
- An activity booklet—to enable you to relate the theory to your own professional knowledge base and work experience.
- A reader, providing key research papers, expert committees' recommendations, articles which develop the concepts underlying the approaches to coronary heart disease risk, accounts of existing schemes, and strategies for risk factor assessment and management.
- An audio cassette which examines patients' experiences of coronary heart disease, their attitudes and health beliefs concerning the causes of coronary heart disease and what can be done to minimise their risks.

The group study pack (£95.00) contains:
- All the above plus
- A video cassette.
- Group leader's notes.

It is also possible to undertake via the Open University certain of their degree-level 9-month courses without enrolment as an undergraduate student.

Further information is available from the Open University, whose address is at the end of the book.

CHAPTER 12

But It's Not Like That at All . . .

Well, perhaps it's not. All this book can do is to give a very middle-of-the-road version of what you are likely to find if you look at the various nursing specialties.

Methods of practice vary as widely as the people who do the job—and some do it more effectively than others. Unless you are enthusiastic about the job you choose and feel it is worth while, then you are unlikely to do it very well.

All I can hope to do is to give you the opportunity to choose your own path from a base of some understanding of what it may entail—and perhaps to emphasise yet again that your future, and thus the progress of the profession, is in your hands. Go for it. Good luck!

Useful Addresses

Government departments

Department of Education and Science
Awards Branch
Government Buildings
Honeypot Lane
Stanmore
Middlesex HA7 1AZ

Telephone number: 01–928 9222

Department of Health and Social Security
Alexander Fleming House
Elephant and Castle
London SE1 6TE

Telephone number: 01–407 5522

Department of Health and Social Security (Northern
    Ireland)
Dundonald House
Upper Newtownards Road
Belfast BT4 3SF

Telephone number: 0232 650111

National Health Service Training Authority
St Bartholomew's Court
18 Christmas Street
Bristol BS1 5BT

Telephone number: 0272 291029

Scottish Home and Health Department
St Andrews House
Edinburgh BH1 3DH

Telephone number: 031–556 8501

Welsh Office Health and Social Work Department
Crown Offices
Cathays Park
Cardiff CF1 3NQ

Telephone number: 0222 825111

Statutory bodies for nursing

English National Board for Nursing, Midwifery and
    Health Visiting
Victory House
170 Tottenham Court Road
London W1P 0HA

Telephone number: 01–388 3131

National Board for Nursing, Midwifery and Health
    Visiting for Northern Ireland
RAC House
79 Chichester Street
Belfast BT1 4JE

Telephone number: 0232 238152

National Board for Nursing, Midwifery and Health
    Visiting for Scotland
22 Queen Street
Edinburgh EH2 1JX

Telephone number: 031–226 7371

Northern Ireland Health and Social Services Training
  Board
The Beeches
Hampton Park
Belfast BT7 3JN

Telephone number: 0232 644811

United Kingdom Central Council for Nursing, Midwifery
  and Health Visiting
23 Portland Place
London W1A 1BA

Telephone number: 01–637 7181

Welsh National Board for Nursing, Midwifery and
  Health Visiting
Floor 13
Pearl Assurance House
Greyfriars Road
Cardiff CF1 3AG

Telephone number: 0222 395535

Other addresses

Association of Commonwealth Universities
John Foster House
36 Gordon Square
London WC1H 0PF

Telephone number: 01–387 8572

Association of Radical Midwives
8A The Drive
Wimbledon
London SW20 (letters only)

Central Register and Clearing House Ltd
c/o English National Board
Victory House
170 Tottenham Court Road
London W1P 0HA (letters only)

Community Mental Handicap Nurses Association
28 Pendlebury Road
Swinton
Manchester M27 1AR (letters only)

Community Psychiatric Nurses Association
c/o H. Rankin
Gloucester House
Southmead Hospital
Westbury on Trym
Bristol BS10 5NB (letters only)

Continuing Nurse Education Programme
26 Danbury Street
London N1 8JU

Telephone number: 01–354 3718

Council for National Academic Awards
344–354 Grays Inn Road
London WC1X 8PT

Telephone number: 01–278 4411

Distance Learning Centre
South Bank Polytechnic
PO Box 310
London SW4 9RZ

Telephone number: 01–228 2015

District Nursing Association
57 Lower Belgrave Street
London SW1W 0LR

Telephone number: 01–730 0110

District Nursing Association (Scotland)
26 Castle Terrace
Edinburgh EH1 2EL

Telephone number: 031–229 7717

English National Board Careers Advisory Centre
PO Box 356
Sheffield S8 0SJ

Telephone number: 0742 551064

Health Visitors Association
36 Eccleston Square
London SW1V 1PF

Telephone number: 01–834 9523

Institute of Health Service Administrators
75 Portland Place
London W1N 4AN

Telephone number: 01–580 5041

Institute of Personnel Management
35 Camp Road
London SW19

Telephone number: 01–946 9100

Open University
Walton Hall
Milton Keynes
MK7 6AA

Telephone number: 0908 653743 (and check your
telephone directory for the nearest regional office)

Polytechnics Central Admissions System
PO Box 67
Cheltenham
Gloucestershire GL50 3AP

Telephone number: 0242 526225

Queen's Nursing Institute
57 Lower Belgrave Square
London SW1W 0LR

Telephone number: 01–730 0355

Radical Health Visitors Group
c/o BSSRS
9 Poland Street
London W1V 3DG (letters only)

Royal College of Midwives
15 Mansfield Street
London W1M 0BE

Telephone number: 01–580 6523

Royal College of Nursing
20 Cavendish Square
London W1M 0AB

You should address enquiries to the appropriate
department:
Community Nursing Association

Daphne Heald Research and Development Unit
Institute of Advanced Nursing Education
Research Society
Society of Mental Handicap Nursing
Society of Occupational Health Nursing
Society of Psychiatric Nursing
etc.

Telephone number: 01—409 3333

Royal College of Nursing (Northern Ireland Board)
17 Windsor Avenue
Belfast BT9 6BE

Telephone number: 0232 668236

Royal College of Nursing (Scottish Board)
44 Heriot Row
Edinburgh EH3 6EV

Telephone number: 031—225 7231

Royal College of Nursing (Welsh Board)
Ty Maeth
King George V Drive East
Cardiff CF4 4XZ

Telephone number: 0222 751373

Scottish Health Visitors Association
47 Timber Bush
Leith
Edinburgh EH6 6QH

Telephone number: 031—553 5233

Universities Central Council on Admissions
PO Box 28
Cheltenham
Gloucestershire GL50 1HY (letters only)

University of London
Department of Extra-Mural Studies
26 Russell Square
London WC1B 5DQ (letters only)

Further reading

Journals

Health Service Journal, Macmillan Magazines Ltd.
Health Visitor, Health Visitors Association.
International Journal of Nursing Studies, Pergamon
  Press.
International Nursing Review, International Council of
  Nurses.
Journal of Advanced Nursing, Blackwell.
Journal of District Nursing, PTM Publishers Ltd.
Lampada, Scutari Projects Ltd for the Royal College of
  Nursing.
Nurse Education Today, Churchill Livingstone.
Nursing Standard, Scutari Projects Ltd.
Nursing Times (with *Community Outlook*), Macmillan
  Magazines Ltd.
Primary Health Care, Scutari Projects Ltd.
Professional Nurse, Austen Cornish Publishers.
Senior Nurse, Blackwell.

Viewing

A Way of Thinking. Video on post-basic nursing
opportunities in both VHS and Betamax, DHSS.

Reference books

*Directory of First Degree and Diploma of Higher
  Education Courses* (annual), Council for National
  Academic Awards.
English National Board publications: for a full list of the
  English National Board publications, which include
  the syllabuses of many of the courses mentioned in
  this book, write to the English National Board for

Nursing, Midwifery and Health Visiting at the address given on p. 112.

Handbook of Degree and Advanced Courses, National Association of Teachers in Further and Higher Education.

Directory of Schools of Medicine and Nursing (annual), Kogan Page.

Hospitals and Health Service Yearbook (annual), Institute of Health Service Management.

Institute of Advanced Education Prospectus (annual), Royal College of Nursing.

Schedule of Postgraduate Courses in UK Universities (annual), Association of Commonwealth Universities.

Directory of Nursing Scholarships, Bursaries and Grants, Royal College of Nursing.

Index